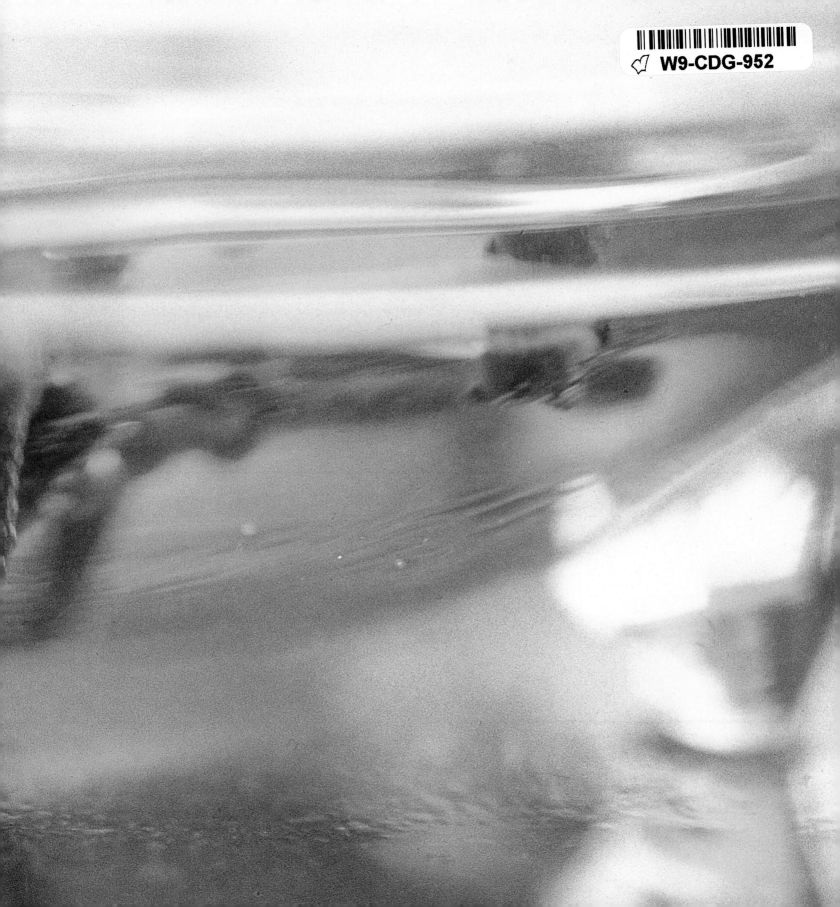

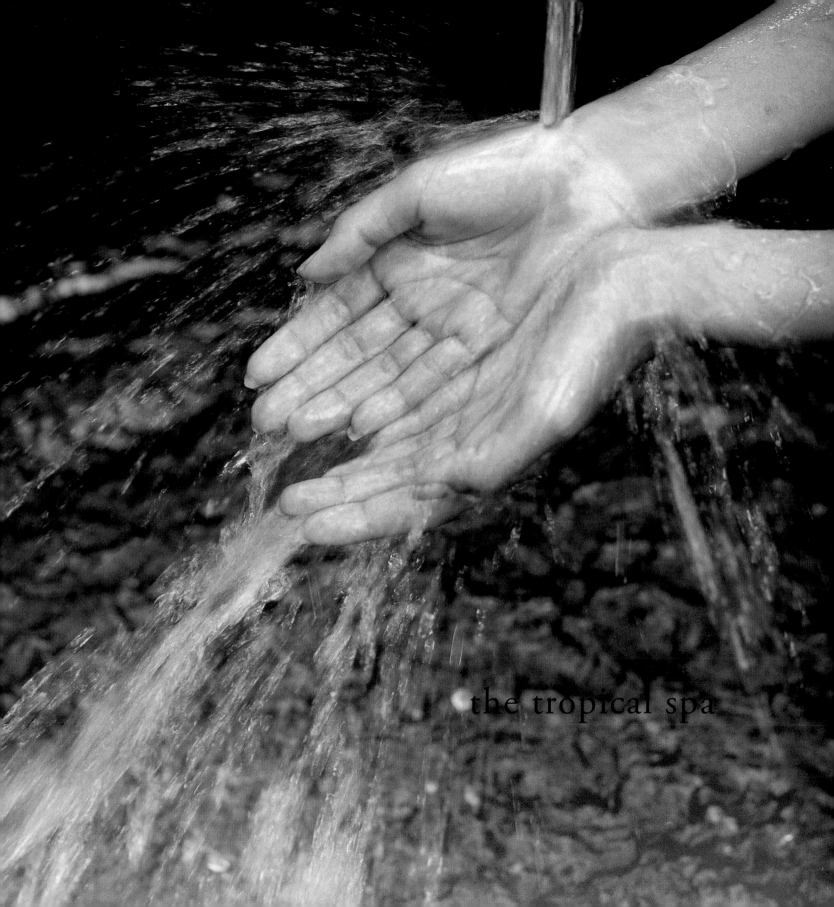

the tropical spa

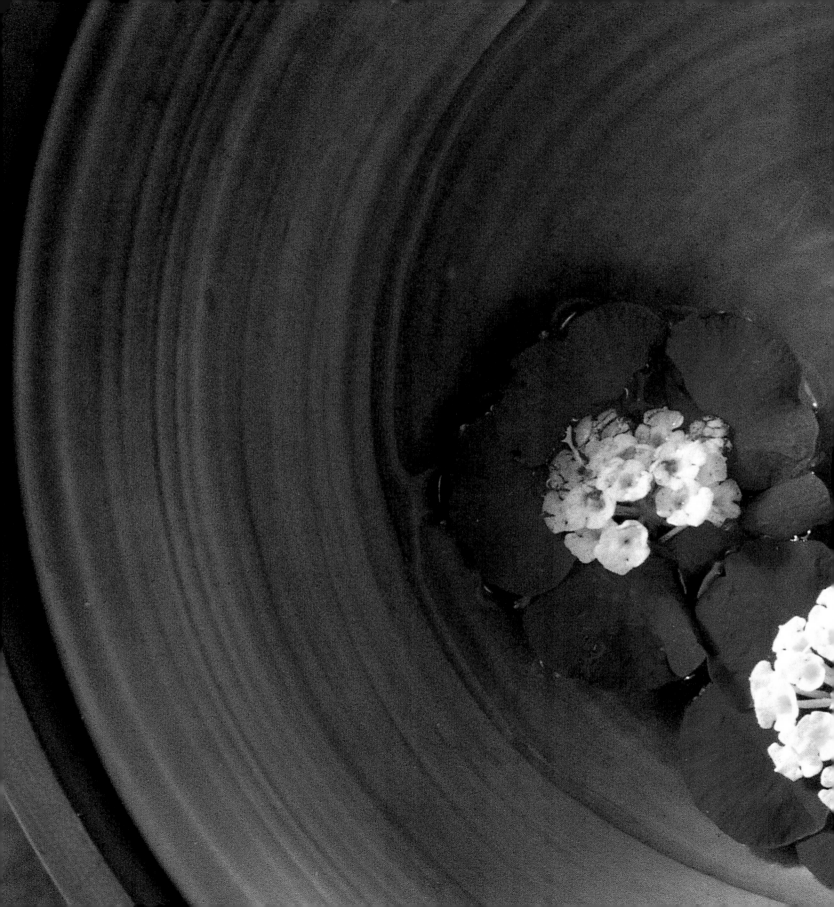

the tropical spa

Asian secrets of health, beauty and relaxation

By Sophie Benge
Photos by Luca Invernizzi Tettoni

PERIPLUS

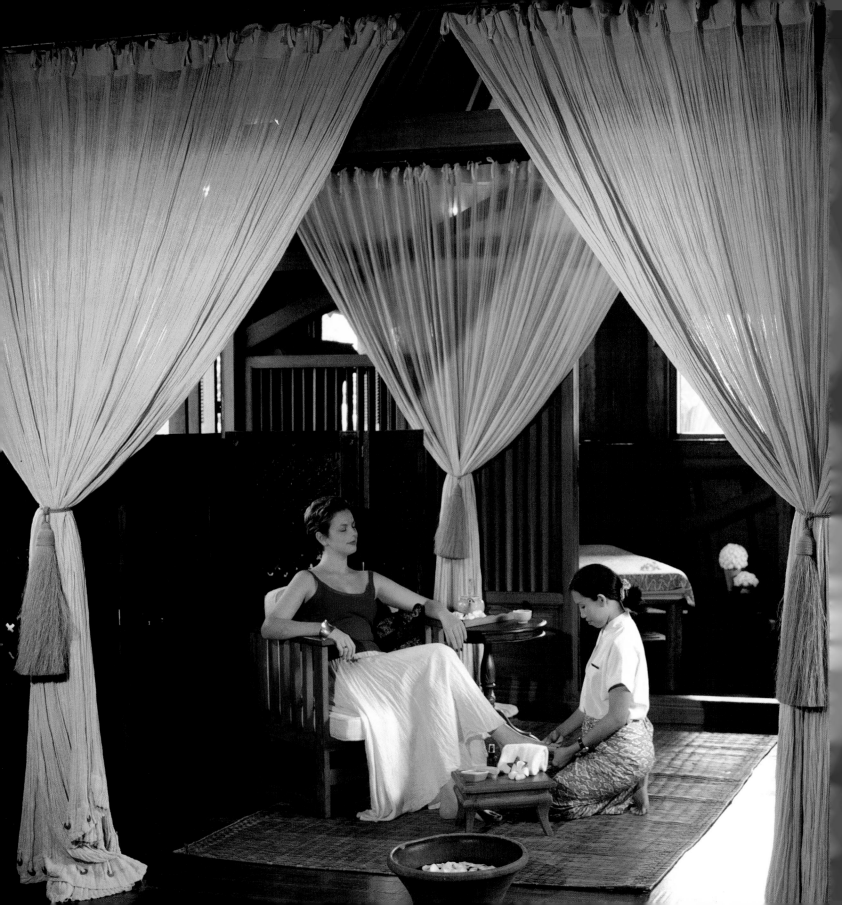

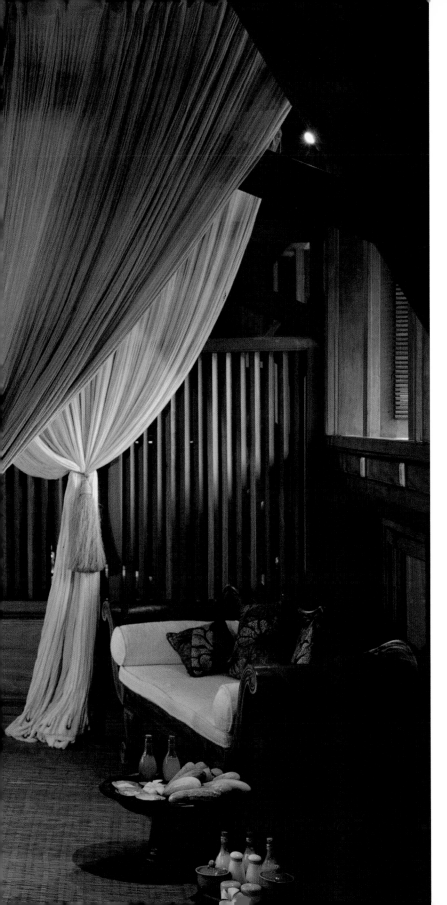

The Tropical Spa
Asian Secrets of Health, Beauty and Relaxation

Published by Periplus Editions (HK) Ltd
Copyright © 1999 Periplus Editions (HK) Ltd

Publisher: Eric Oey
Associate Publisher: Christina Ong
Editor: Kim Inglis
Designer: Loretta Reilly

ISBN 962–593–265–8

Distributed by:
Tuttle Publishing (USA)
264 Innovation Drive
North Clarendon
VT 065759–9700
Toll-free order number: 1–800–526–2778

Berkeley Books Pte Ltd (Asia Pacific)
5 Little Road, #08–01
Singapore 536983
Tel 65 280–1330

Tuttle Publishing (Japan)
RK Building, 2nd Floor
2–13–10 Shimo-Meguro
Meguro-ku
Tokyo 1530064
Tel 81 3 5437–0171

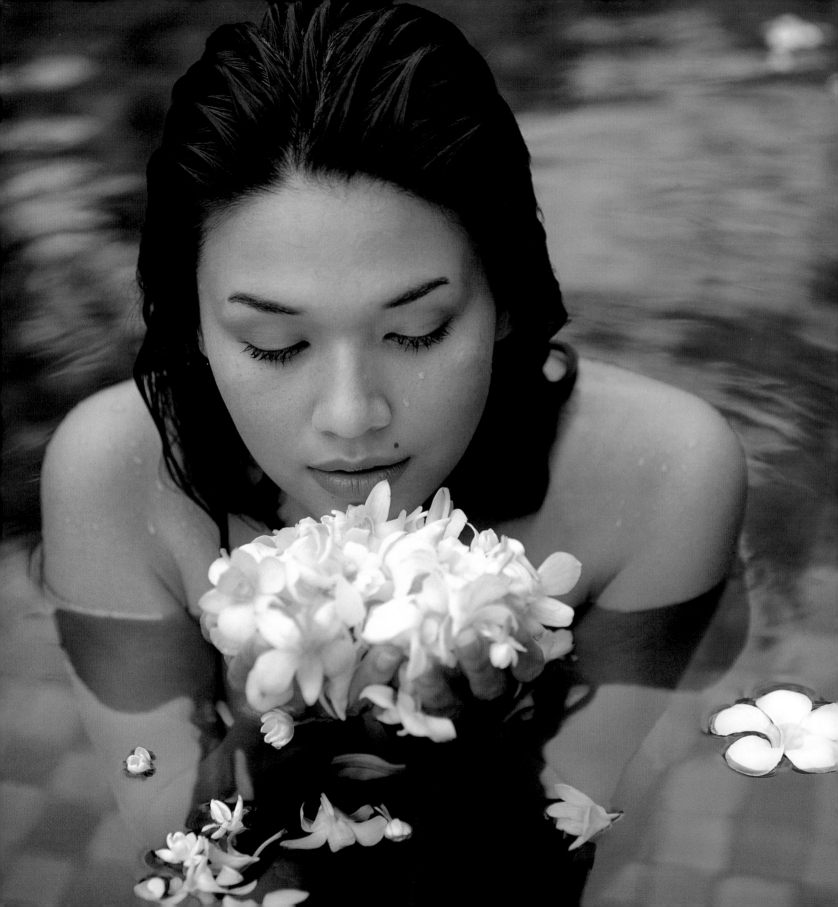

contents

8

The Tropical Spa Experience

Living the spa life: an introduction to the roots of Asian beauty, the history of traditional, natural treatments and therapies, and how they are offered in a tropical spa setting.

22

Top Tropical Spas

Banyan Tree Spa Phuket, 24
Banyan Tree Spa Bintan, 26
The Source at Begawan Giri Estate, 28
Mandara Spa at The Chedi, 32
Chiva-Som, 36
Mandara Spa at The Datai, 40
The Spa at Jimbaran, Four Seasons Resort, 42
Spa at Bali Hyatt, 46
Mandara Spa at the Ibah, 50
Nirwana Spa at Le Meridien Bali, 54
The Nusa Dua Spa, 56
The Oriental Spa, 60
The Pita Maha Private Villa Spa, 64
Spa at Hotel Tugu, 66

70

Asian Health and Beauty Secrets

Body Conscious, 72
Rites of Massage, 96
Mind–Body–Spirit, 110
Face Value, 118
Hair Story, 128
Feet First, 138

148

Asian Spa Cuisine

A Kickstart to the Day, 150
Simple Food, 152
A Natural Feast, 154
Tasteful Thai, 156
Dining Light, 158
Liquid Assets, 160
Herbal Tonics, 162
Cooking with Condiments, 164

166

Natural Spa Ingredients, 166
Natural Spa Products, 172
Resource and Spa Directories, 175

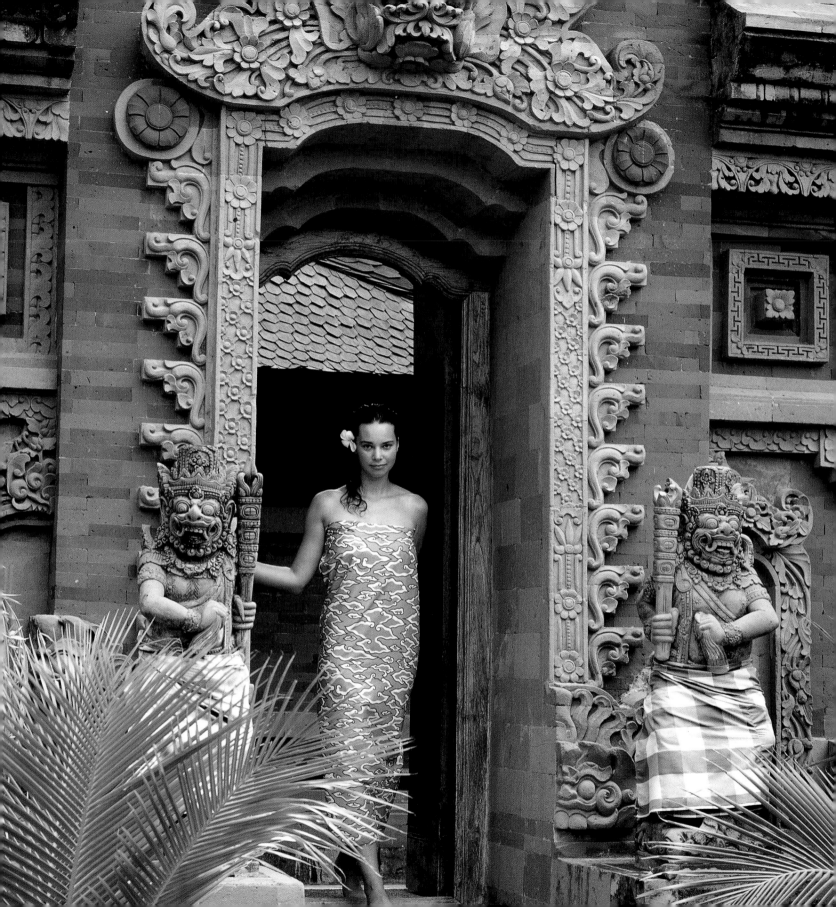

the tropical spa experience

'Spa' is the Millennium buzzword for health, beauty and relaxation; it is hip in holiday-speak and a mantra for the growing band of worshippers at the altar of self-preservation. Yet despite its current popularity in the lives of trendsetters, jet setters and health fanatics everywhere, the 'spa' is not a new stop on the road to wellbeing. It is a concept as old as the hills it springs from, rewritten for the contemporary scene.

In broad terms, this new image has developed to meet the prevailing mood for an holistic approach to life. In today's era of 'mindfulness', the pursuit of vanity and pampering is happily fused with a desire for inner health. Destination spas, mushrooming on every continent, set out to offer some solutions for those who want to look good, feel good and rejuvenate their bodies as well as their souls.

This is an extension of the original spa concept which, although it has existed since Roman times, was only formalized in 17th-century Europe out of an understanding for the curative powers of water. The spa, such as the eponymous resort in Belgium or the historical Baden-Baden in Germany, originated as a clinical, get-well centre for curing all manner of diseases from arthritis to infertility. Rigorous routines, in often less than indulgent locations, involved drinking or bathing in the spring-fed spa waters or walking barefoot in the winter dew at dawn.

Today, the spa philosophy has moved on from the pain-is-gain approach and away from a curative emphasis towards a preventive one.

And while there are country by country variations in the spa experience (for example, the emphasis in the United States is not in any way self-indulgent), the cutting edge is the Orient with its focus on spiritual harmony and natural, not pharmaceutical or clinical, treatments. The irony is that a spa culture is not traditional to tropical Asia: yet the centuries-old health and beauty practices of this region are being picked up and repackaged for spa retreats from California to Kensington.

The tropical or southeast Asian health and beauty philosophy stands in stark contrast to traditional Western beliefs that put faith in the contents of a gold-topped tub or in the hands of white-coated laboratory technologists. Year after year, the bible for beauticians across Europe and America has preached skin deep remedies, from wrinkle-reduction creams to liposuction, for the ultimate in cover girl glamour. It is, however, a relatively recent revelation that beauty from the outside in is back to the front. Now it is more a case of a leg wax plus a dose of soul nourishment, please, for today's 'mindful' and rejuvenating treatment.

(Page 4–5) The exclusive one-villa spa at the Ibah in Bali is spacious and decorated like a luxurious home, just as the owners of this enchanting hotel wanted. As a result, it offers one of the most rarefied and personal spa experiences in Bali.

(Previous page) One of the appealing aspects of the Tropical Spa is the floral heaven that goes with it. Frangipani and jasmine blooms are never out of sight in Asia and their aromas must be among the sweetest of all tropical flowers.

< The *Bali Padma* uses traditional stonecarving throughout the spa premises.

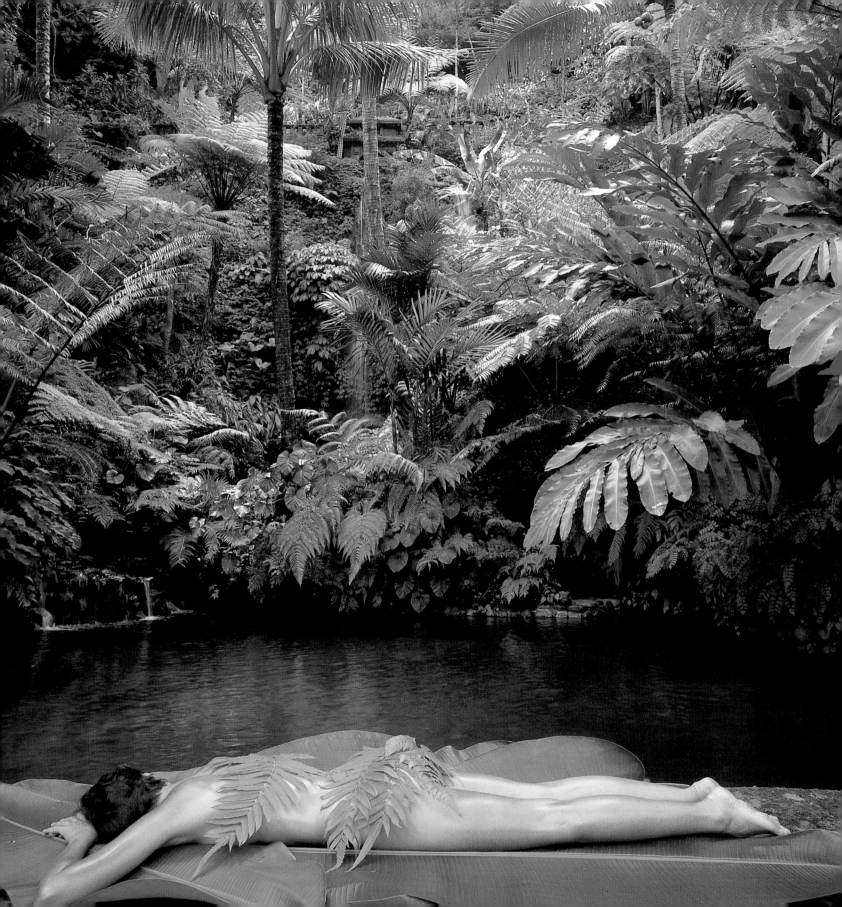

"The mind and the body are like parallel universes. Anything that happens in the mental universe, must leave tracks in the physical one." *Deepak Chopra*

This worldwide vogue for spiritual and mental, as well as physical, fitness has been at the core of Asian beauty custom since the beginning of time. Lasting beauty comes from deep within the body and mind; how we feel about ourselves and the world around us directly affects our facial expression and outward appearance. Modern mind-body science has now shown that when we are relaxed and happy, the biochemical rhythms in our bodies are significantly different to those present when we are angry, tense or sad. In his best seller, *Quantum Healing*, celebrity physician and mind-body guru, Deepak Chopra, writes: "…the mind and the body are like parallel universes. Anything that happens in the mental universe, must leave tracks in the physical one."

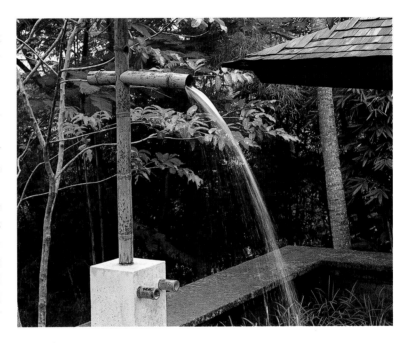

In Indonesia, the birthplace of many tropical health and beauty secrets, there is an ancient Javanese expression: *rupasampat wahya bhiantara*, – which encapsulates exactly this notion. It roughly translates as 'the balance between inner and outer beauty, between that which is visible and that which lies within' and it is the parable by which women in this part of the world live without even thinking about it.

According to Dr Martha Tilaar, the founder and president of one of the country's fore-most natural cosmetic groups, outer beauty involves a ritualistic process using natural products for skin, hair and body. This is balanced by a number of inner beauty techniques, which include taking jamu (traditional herbal tonics and medicines); practising *Daya Putih*, a spiritual form of exercise which unleashes inner power to maintain purity; fasting; and making more frequent giving, selfless gestures in our lives. "A sense of gratitude and taking care of others," she explains, "empowers us inside. This is not religious practice; it is all part of beauty ritual."

< *The Source at Begawan Giri Estate* has taken the outdoor spa concept to its ultimate, natural conclusion.

^ The outdoor shower, such as this one at *Begawan Giri* is synonymous with the Tropical Spa.

" To twist and…stretch is…a body holiday. There is the unexpected delight in meeting earth and sky at the same moment! Gravity." From *Awakening the Spine – A New Way of Yoga* by Vanda Scaravelli

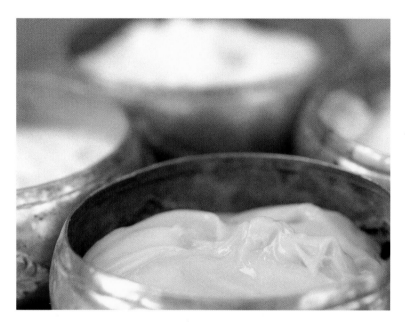

mindful movement, there are other more familiar routes such as the soft exercise techniques of yoga, meditation, *tai chi* and *qi gong*. In practising these oriental art forms, which concentrate our attention on breathing and body rhythms, we can go a long way toward clearing our minds from daily dross and becoming aware of our mind-body interdependence.

What this enlightened subterfuge means in plain English is that these forms of gentle exercise do as much for easing tension as treatments themselves. And a relaxed state of mind enables clarity of thought, which in turn, enhances beauty. Again, Deepak Chopra stresses the importance of meditation: "To make the right choices in life, you have to get in touch with your soul. To do this you need to experience solitude, which most people are afraid of because in the silence you hear the truth and know the solution. Ultimately the only solution to all problems are spiritual."

Besides meditation and yogic exercise, a unique way of getting in touch with our spiritual souls (female only) is available at Naz Workshops, Singapore. Trained aromatherapist and horticulturist Nazli Anwari and her partner Cheyenne Goh are aiming to give back to south-east Asian women a part of their heritage in the form of their interactive 'Erotic Women's Workshops' based on aromatherapy and Asian

∧ The crème bath is a ubiquitous hair product in Asia. It contributes to the sleek shiny locks that women from this region are renowned for.

> Mindful exercise is integral to the Asian spa philosophy. Even though it is in the heart of Bangkok, *The Oriental Spa* is an outpost of serenity, ideal for some meditative moments.

It is also part of the Asian ideology that says that a desire to be beautiful is valid; it is not the vacuous pursuit of vanity that tends to be associated with beauty practices in the West. In his treatise *Daya Putih for the Inner Beauty*, the *Daya Putih* foundation's leader, Sumadi Kertonegro, makes the lofty claim that 'the path to beauty is the path towards consciousness and the origin and purpose of life'.

While Kertonegro's path to beauty and life's purpose is through the spiritual patterns of *Daya Putih*, which claims that the Hindu gods dwell in our body's organs and must be assuaged through

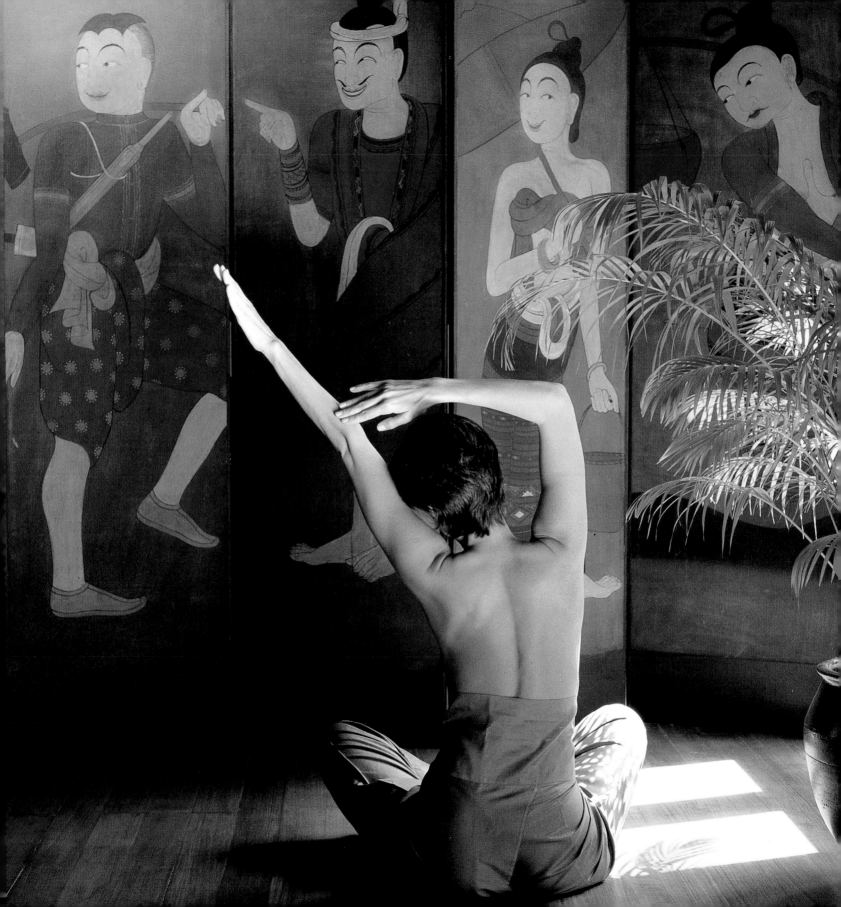

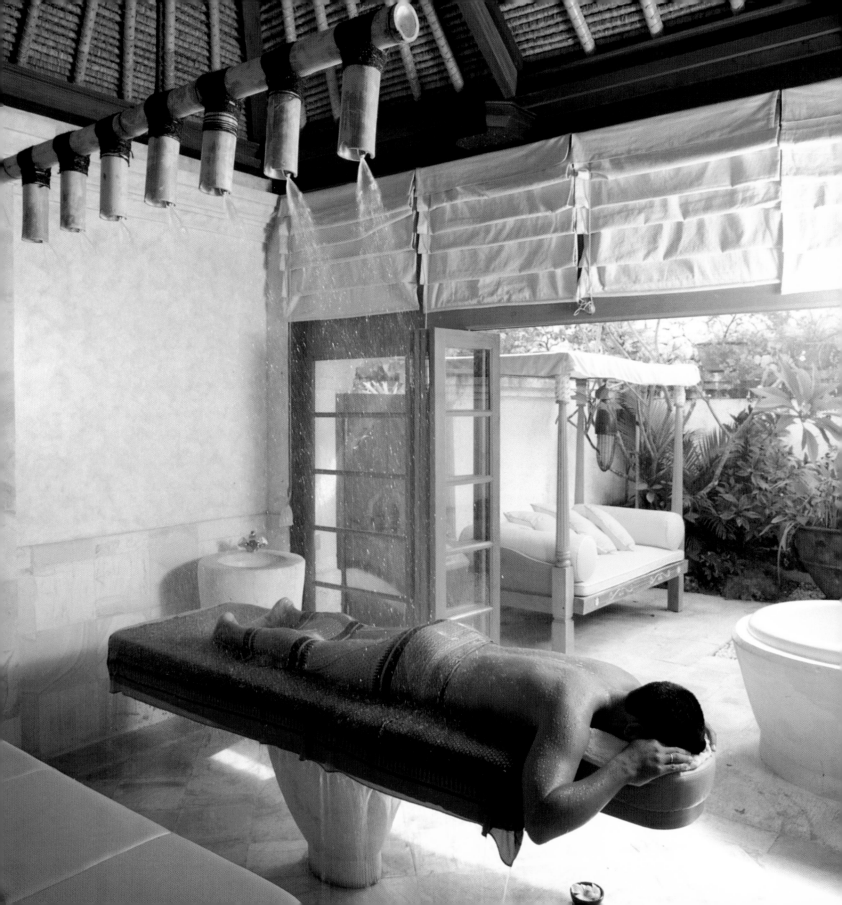

"Women today are losing their vital force. Even their posture says, 'I don't feel great any more.' We help them get back in touch with their sensuality." – *Nazli Anwari*

herbs. Says Anwari, "Women today are losing their vital force. Even their posture says, 'I don't feel great any more.'"We help them get back in touch with their sensuality." In the belief that there is an alchemist in us all, these workshops encourage women to mix herbs and spices to make their own body scrubs, to blend their own floral oils, to make herbal tea infusions and their own floral cleansing waters. In this way they are getting back in touch with nature. Also by learning to massage themselves and by taking time to soak in a flower bath, they are getting back in touch with their bodies – a sensual, rewarding ritual that Anwari believes plays little if no role in women's lives today.

All of this could be described as humanizing herbs and spices. But whatever guise you choose, the focus on nature's store cupboard and her rich aromas is giving Asian beauty worldwide appeal. Leaf shampoos, crushed nut conditioners and cocounut body scrubs fall in line with the new mood for 'eco-chic', where eco-consciousness and style are no longer mutually exclusive.

While a deepening commitment to environmental consumerism now grips the West, it has been the mainstay of Asian culture until recent economic development. In the realm of health and beauty, answers to radiant skin, shiny hair and cures for cancer have been found in the

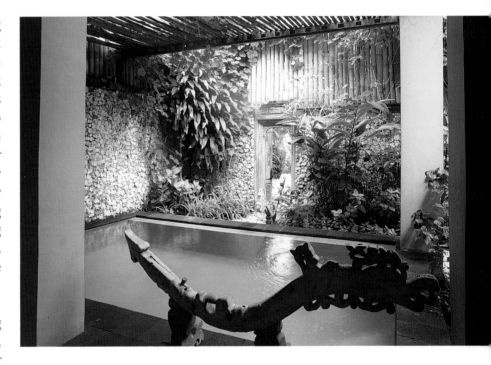

region's vast botanical heritage. On the Indonesian island of Java alone, 6,500 species of plant, 4,500 of which are native to Java, have been recorded. Malaysia lays claim to 3,600 species of tree, and other tracts of rain forest in the region still wait to be discovered.

Many of the natural treatments that are now commonly used throughout tropical Asian countries trace their origins to the palaces of Central Java. From the 17th century until today, princesses from the *keratons* of Solo, Yogyakarta

< The *Spa at Jimbaran* is the only tropical spa where you can take a shower lying down. These jets replicate rainfall to send you into a relaxed state.

∧ An entity unto itself! The *Spa at Hotel Tugu* is truly 'traditional', with barely a hint of 20th-century trappings.

"Whosoever offers me with devotion a leaf, a flower, a fruit or water, that offering of love, of the pure heart, I accept." *From the 'Mahabharata'; the god Krishna explains what God expects of an offering.*

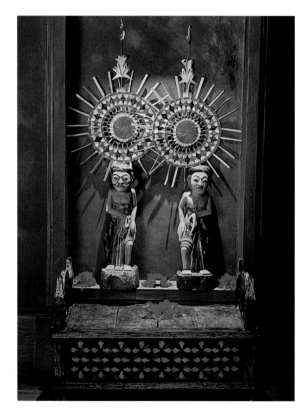

Ibu Mooryati Soedibyo is a princess-turned-business woman who has adapted much of the royal heritage she learnt in the *keraton* as a child into one of Indonesia's biggest beauty businesses manufacturing traditional cosmetics under the Mustika Ratu name. Soedibyo remembers her disciplined Javanese upbringing, which taught her how to weave her hair with pandanus leaves as a young girl and how to make a *ukel* (outsized hairpiece) from her own locks. She made her own shampoo, by burning rice stalks and soaking them in water until they turned into a sticky ash paste, and her own face powder by personally grinding *bengkuang* and turmeric roots with rice. Now in her seventies, her 60-year relationship with a natural pharmacopoeia has done her visibly proud.

It is the fairytale quality of experiences such as those of Ibu Mooryati that have lent the Asian beauty boom its allure and mystique. One of its most important aspects which has long been exported to other cultures, is its concentration on the healing and soothing powers of massage. The tactile sense is an unquestioned part of life in many parts of Asia; people carry compassion in their hands, which they transmit as a matter of course. "It is like being nurtured by our mothers," says spa consultant Dorinda Rose Berry. "People need that unconditional love in their lives which are so full of gadgets and computers. We no longer need material things, we just need love."

and Surakarta experimented with natural potions and lotions, concocted by themselves. Some secret remedies are still kept under wraps behind palace walls; others, such as the Javanese Lulur, have found their way around the region, even around the world. This famous body scrub of rice, spices and splashes of natural yoghurt is a skin softening elixir set to beat the best designer bubbles and moisturizing body creams money can buy.

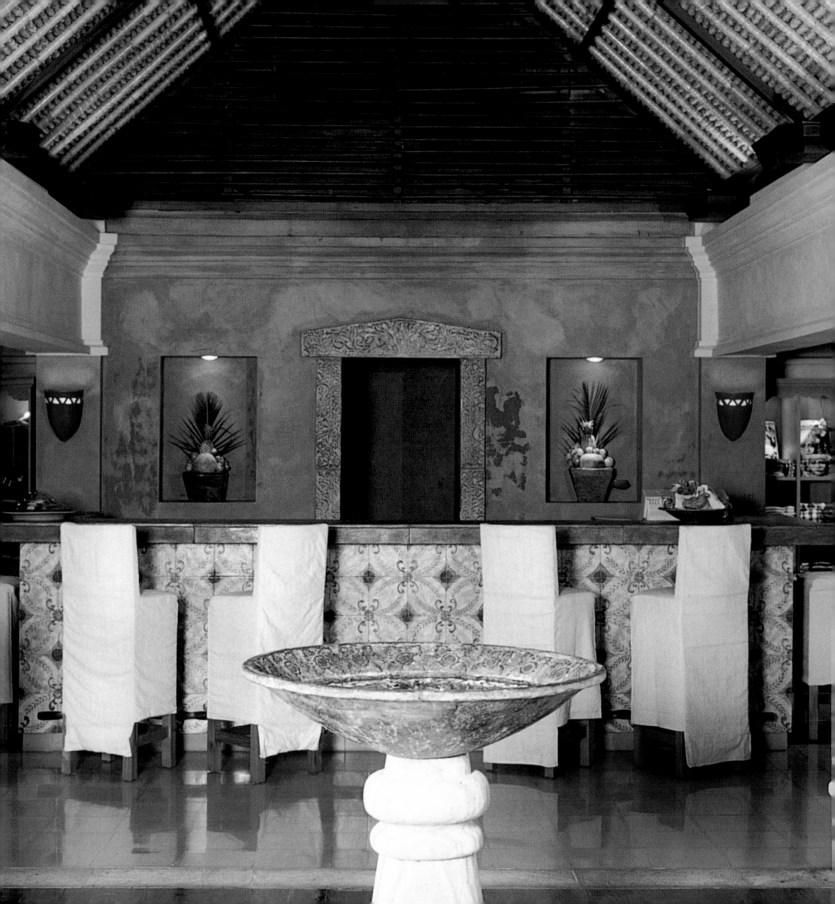

"Thai massage is a healing experience for the giver as well as the receiver and intrinsic life energy will flow between the two." *Khun Sutthichai Teimeesak, chief massage therapist at the Oriental Spa, Bangkok*

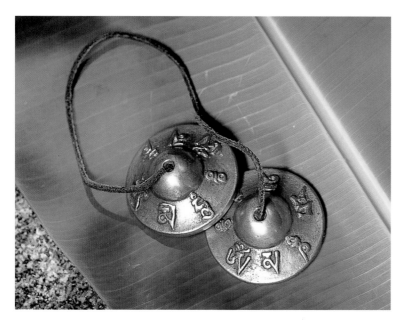

∧ These *ching* (chimes) are used in Thai folk dance and music festivals. At *Banyan Tree Spa Phuket*, their delicate sound is often heard wafting through the silence.

＞ Outdoor massage, such as here at *Chiva-Som*, Thailand, is high on the Tropical Spa agenda.

The tropical spa experience is based on un-conditional love as much as, if not more than, anything else. The notion that weary souls can receive compassionate care and attention without payback goes a long way to explaining why they are so popular. Spa therapists make their clients feel special which, coming from their fast-paced situations at home, is exactly what they crave. They also want time out, but they want more than the standard two weeks of poolside lounging. Serenity, soul-soothing and stress-busting is what they're after and the tropical spa knows how to provide it, some argue, better than any other type of spa retreat.

At the tropical spa there is nothing of the continental preference for municipal buildings and matronly Fraus in white coats; none of the fading chintz and timid teenage therapists of the British country house-turned-spa; and no evidence of the seriousness and self-flagellation of the Stateside spa regime. Nor does the tropical spa display any of the glitz and kitsch of those bandwagon spa resorts that are floundering to find their meaning in the world of wellbeing.

As resort companies begin to realize the value of the region's traditions, they are opening an increasing number of tropical spas in the destinations of our dreams. These venues uplift our spirits before we even put one foot into the treatment room. An arduous journey from the Indonesian capital of Jakarta immediately becomes worthwhile on arrival at *Javana Spa* which is set in the foothills of mountainous rain forest, gushing with waterfalls and ringing with the cries of monkeys and birds. The tropical setting with its healing, spring-fed dipping pools, is part of the restorative experience at *Begawan Giri Estate*, Bali. And at the *Novotel Coralia* in Lombok, lie in your own pavilion on an isolated patch of white-sand beach while sea breezes and healing hands stroke your body in time with the sound of the waves on the empty, turquoise sea.

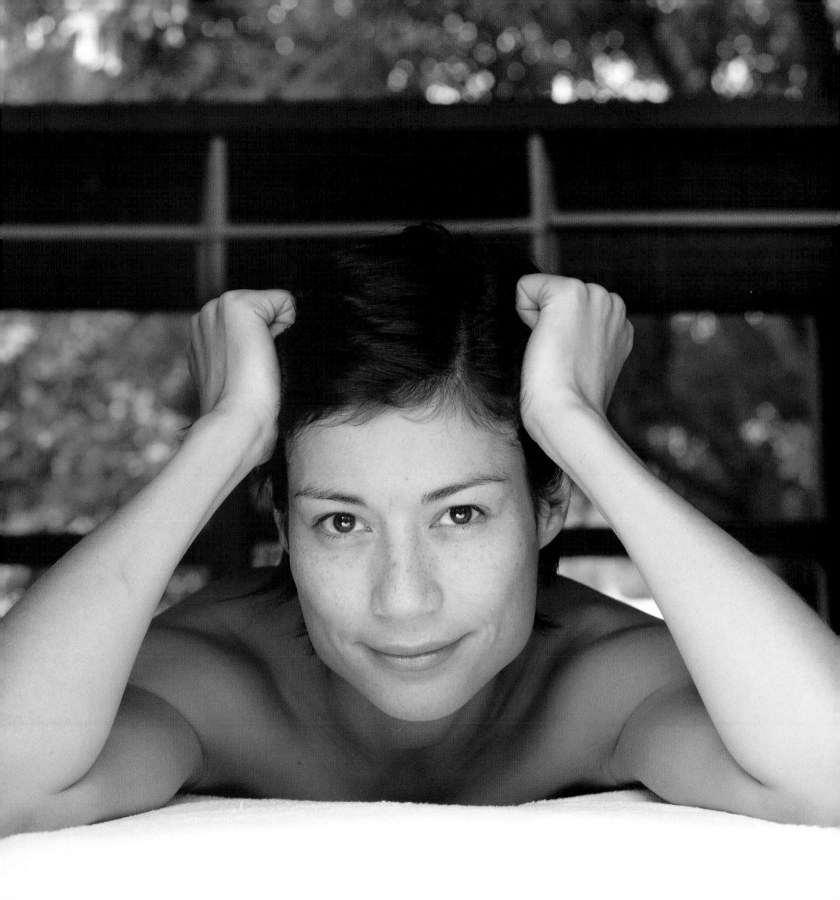

"If you want skin that is irresistible to the touch, the secret is to touch yourself,"
Pratima Raichur, Ayurvedic physician

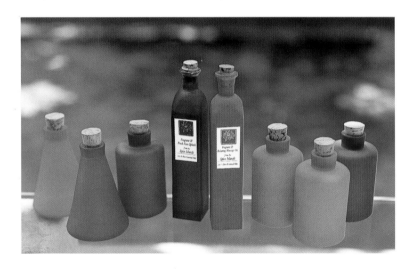

∧ 'Spice Islands'
oils from Esens
are rich in
aromatic scents
and pretty in their
coloured glass
bottles. They are
available at Bali's
Nusa Dua Spa.

(*Overleaf*) The
Nikko stands
proud like a castle
on the southern
tip of Bali's Nusa
Dua peninsula. The
resort's spa is
mapped out like a
village street, with
courtyard houses
as treatment
rooms. It lies just
behind the beach .

It is this ability to commune with abundant nature that puts tropical spas in a league of their own. Treatment rooms in all the better spas effortlessly fuse indoor and outdoor space so that it feels quite normal to be doused with water or rubbed with yoghurt while standing naked under the stars. It is somehow liberating to sit naked in a hot jacuzzi pool which teeters on the lip of a dramatic river gorge while, at the same time, listening to frogs and being tickled by ferns that catch the breeze. And it is a rare bucolic pleasure to lie in an outdoor bath and splatter your body with handfuls of flower heads that float alongside in the water.

The tropical treatment processes themselves unravel yet more exotic sensations. A trickle of cucumber pulp between the toes beats rubbing cream in your heels. The heat of cloves and ginger smeared over your shoulder or the pungent smell of coffee bean wafting up from your cleavage elicits a giggle of decadent delight. Nature's store cupboard is feeding your body, but hey, this is also fun!

While the tropical spa experience falls in line with the current vogue for 'back-to-basics' living, the irony is that these spas, on the whole, are chambers of ethnic chic. They give designers the opportunity to blend the best raw materials – textured teakwood, carved stone, cool ceramic, terrazzo, bamboo and *alang-alang* – in indigenous styles with gratuitous design indulgence.

The holistic approach to life at the tropical spa is where it's at. But most us don't find time to go to the dry cleaners let alone to chant or meditate. We may yearn for a two-hour massage in the increasing number of Day Spas but reality is more like ten minutes in the bathroom with a tub of alternative cosmetic cream called something like 'Peace of Mind'. The tropical spa is the only place that offers the real thing. The *Banyan Tree Spa Phuket* speaks for all its cousins in describing itself as a 'sanctuary of the senses' – a buffer from the outside world that people every-where increasingly want and need.

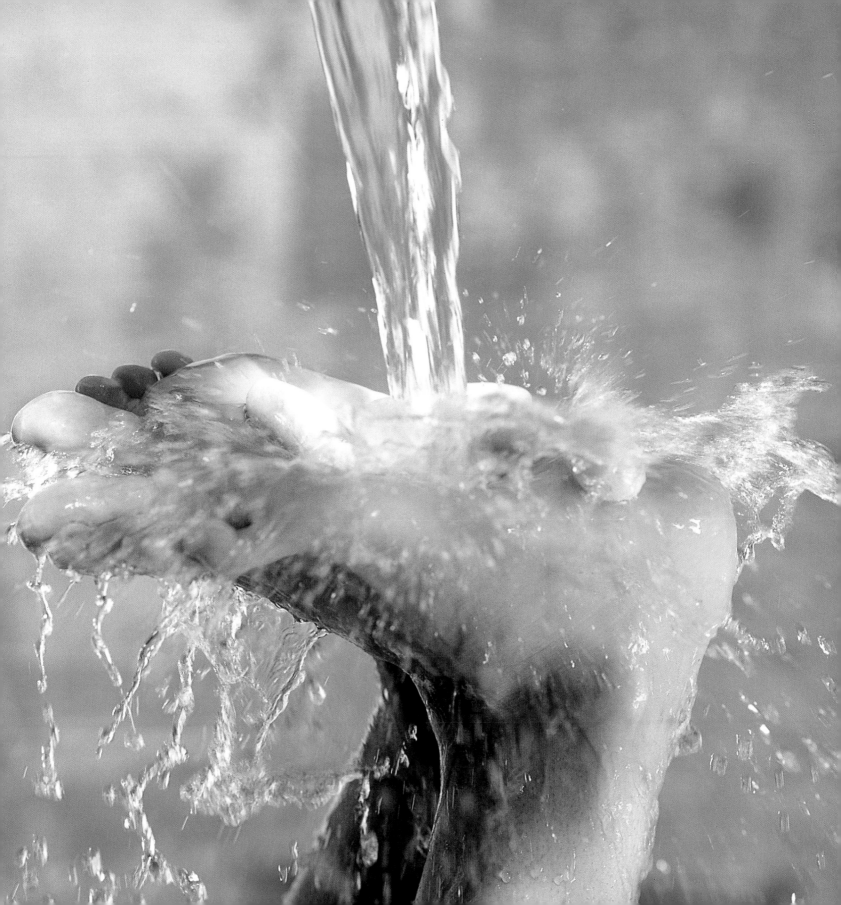

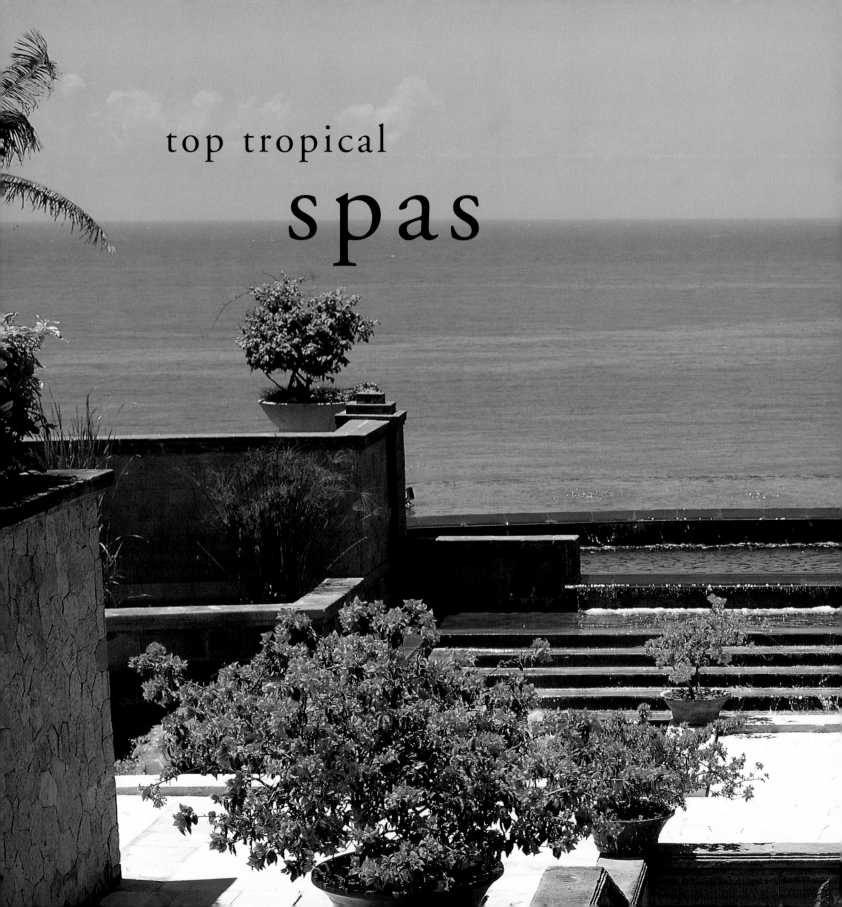

top tropical
spas

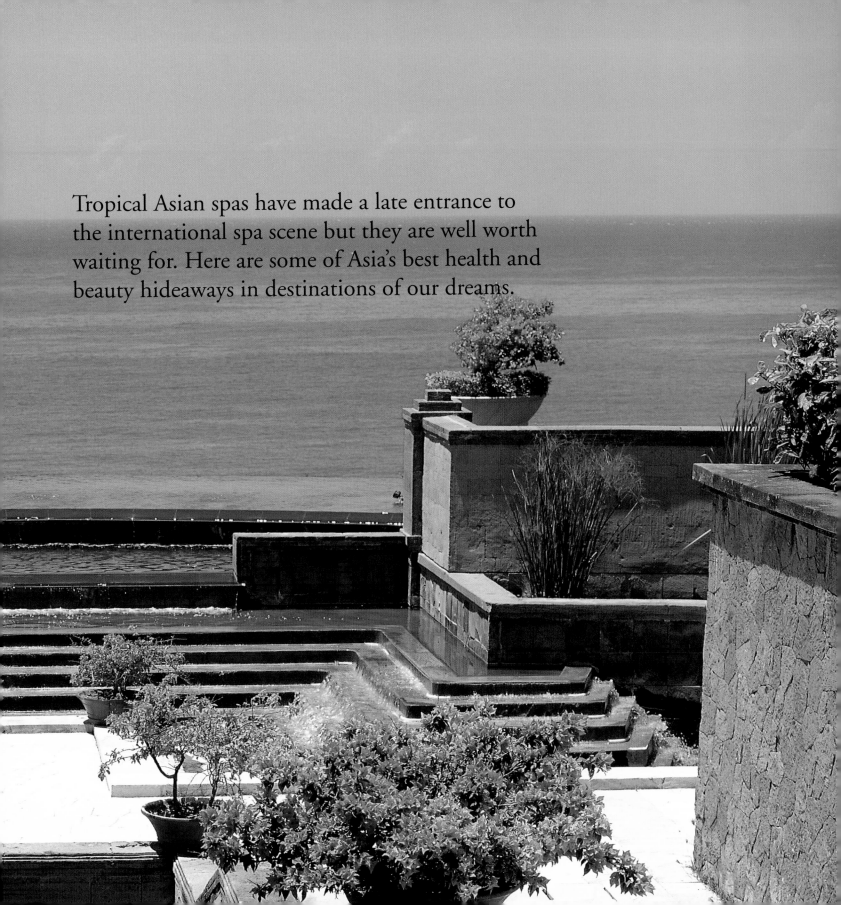

Tropical Asian spas have made a late entrance to the international spa scene but they are well worth waiting for. Here are some of Asia's best health and beauty hideaways in destinations of our dreams.

Banyan Tree Spa Phuket

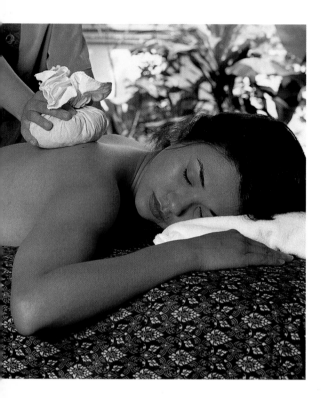

For all the pleasure they lay before you, spas in Asia also present a problem: blood pressure rises in the face of the options on offer. How can the world-weary soul decide between a *Voyage of Peace*, an *Oasis of Bliss* and, for a jet-fresh business man, *The Asian Affair*? Spa goers pour over the treatment menu like it had five stars from Michelin. But in keeping with the Buddhist philosophy that this spa embraces, the *Banyan Tree Spa Phuket* recommends you stick with whatever takes your fancy first. Your intuition will decide what is right for you. It may be honey, mud, sea salt or herbs that are rubbed into your body; but whatever it is, it comes with a little dose of love, the most important ingredient of all.

The people at *Banyan Tree Spa Phuket* believe that love is what is needed most in modern lives that are so alienated by gadgets and material objects. The meditative philosophy and practice of Buddhism (most young men in Thailand spend three months in the monastery as novice monks) allows the Thais (this includes the therapists here) to detach themselves and offer this love unconditionally through their hands. It's not health claims, but relaxation with all her attendant touch, sound, scent and scenery, that is the panacea adopted at this spa.

However, this spa has become so popular that the mood of relaxation can get a little lost in the clamour of souls on its doorstep. Opt for your *Oasis of Bliss* in the privacy of your own Pool Villa, with its extensive proportions, raised *sala* and lap pool within a tropical, walled garden. Here that little extra dose of love, Thai-style, will leave you so relaxed you will never want to leave.

> Each private Pool Villa covers an extraordinary 270 square metres. This nine-metre mini lap pool, as well as the Thai *sala* or outdoor dining area, landscaped gardens and outdoor sunken bath, have all contributed to making the *Banyan Tree Spa Phuket* something of a yardstick among the top-end spa resorts in Asia.

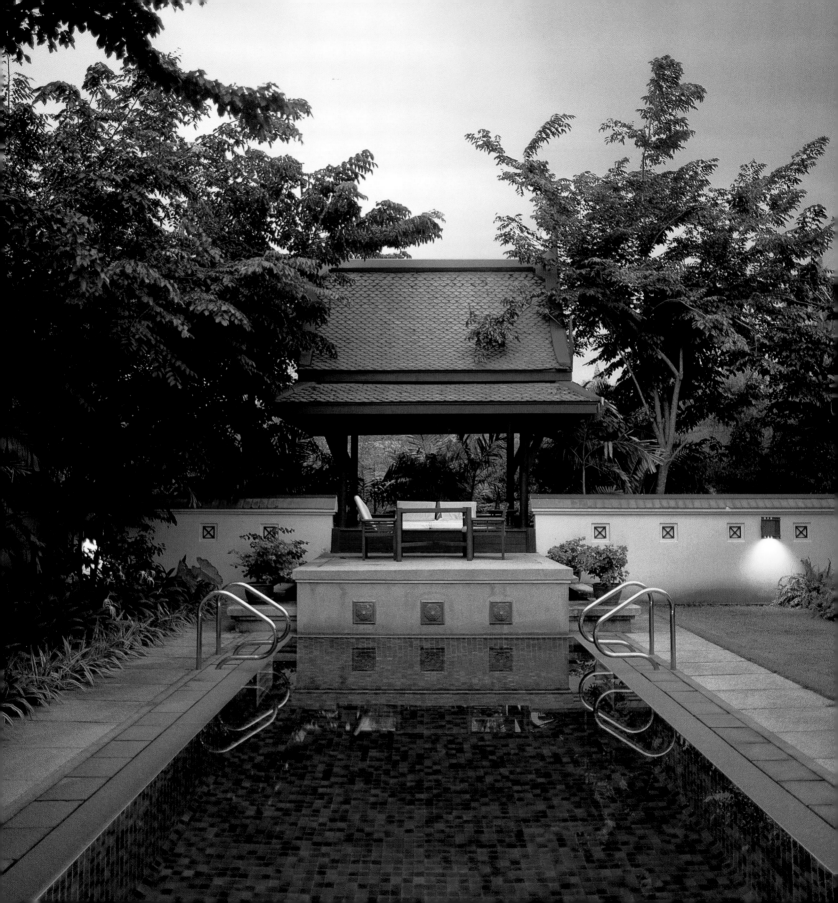

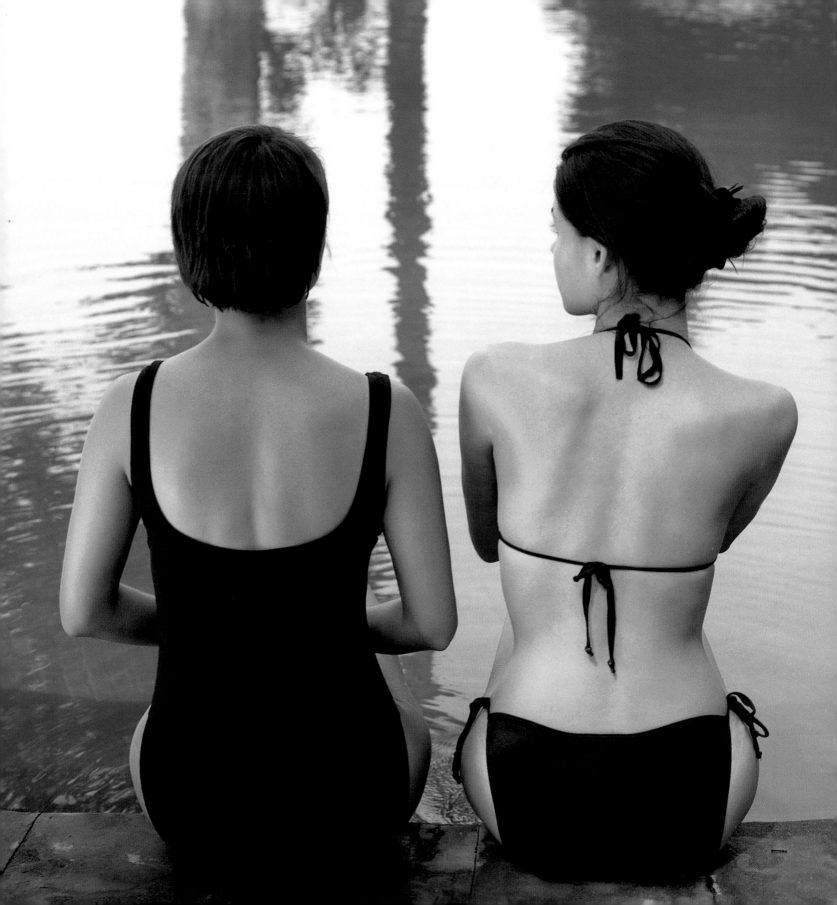

Banyan Tree Spa Bintan

There is little global fanfare about *Banyan Tree Spa Bintan* which is a blessing for those who seek that which has come to classify the essence of an Asian spa resort: tranquillity, therapy and spiritual time out packaged in a tropical setting. *Banyan Tree Spa Bintan* offers it all with understatement.

Perhaps this special little spa misses out on the hype lavished on many of its Asian cousins because it is situated on the relatively unknown Indonesian island of Bintan. Lying just 45 minutes by hydrofoil from Singapore, Bintan is a growing tourist destination with a plethora of new resorts. Never mind; when paddling in a spectacular private villa pool with palm-fringed beach views that sweep to the horizon, who would know that this was not the furthest corner of the South Pacific? And yet it is conveniently located.

The resort's spa pavilion is as tropical as they come, clinging to a cliff face and communing with nature. Watch out for the giant geckos while wending your way along the decking to your treatment room that seems to float over a vociferous ocean below. The nub of the 'tropical spa' assault on the senses lies here in *Banyan Tree Spa Bintan*'s 'Tranquil Room' where the sound is the waves, the view is the seashore, the smell is spicy – burning patchouli, vetiver and clove oils – and the mood is thick with calm. To lay back in here is to let life's pains evaporate from every pore. And then walk along the corridor for a treatment. Otherwise, it's easy to stay in the hilltop villas that are tastefully decorated and feel like home but, undoubtedly, with better views and clean sea breezes.

Treatments here embrace the general gamut of massages, facials and wraps using raw materials and mesmerizing scents, which altogether compound the peaceful experience that this resort already provides.

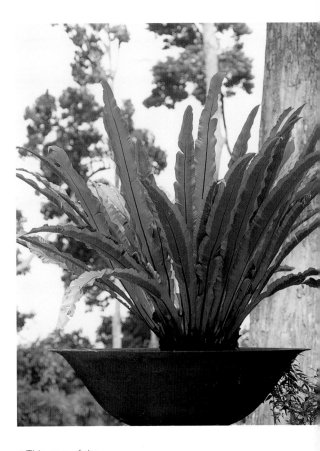

< This, one of the resort's two rock edge swimming pools, overlooks the secluded bay at Tanjong Said, on the northwest tip of Bintan Island.

The Source at Begawan Giri Estate

We have come to associate Bali with the very best in luxury resort hotels, spas and tropical holiday locations so it is something of a feat to have created *Begawan Giri* which outstrips her cousins on so many levels. The nub of her exclusivity – there are only five private residences, each designed to defy description – really lies with her owner. Bradley Gardner has been locked in a passionate clinch with this piece of land ever since he first set foot on its sacred ground over ten years ago. Since then he has fashioned the private estate of his dreams on this extraordinary peninsula.

The spa experience here is an innovative one; it focuses less on passive indulgence and more on guests' ability to tap into their own inner source by embracing the vitality of the landscape. This is not as 'cultish' as it sounds. There is a palpable energy at *Begawan Giri* that flows from a natural spring, revered for miles around for its rejuvenating and healing powers. You don't have to chant mantras to appreciate some meditative moments by one of its natural pools half way down the mountainside above the confluence of two rivers.

The Source, the Estate's 'natural' spa (no spa buildings, receptions or treatment rooms here) is spread all over the estate's eight hectares with walking trails, a 'jungle gym', spring-fed rock pools and outdoor massage pavilions perched among the trees. Restorative programmes – up to three hours long – are conducted in the belief that the body can restore itself with the right kind of guidance: Reiki, meditation, yoga, walking and inner focusing finished off with pampering, all made that much more effective by a setting that is beautifully bewitching.

For the more sedate spa-goer, a full complement of traditional treatments is offered on the decks or in the rooms or poolside of the residences.

> The 'swimming pool' redefined. *Begawan Giri* boasts a number of rock-lined pools fed by water from a holy spring (*see above*). It is said to have inborn healing properties. The pools are always cold, but also chlorine-free.

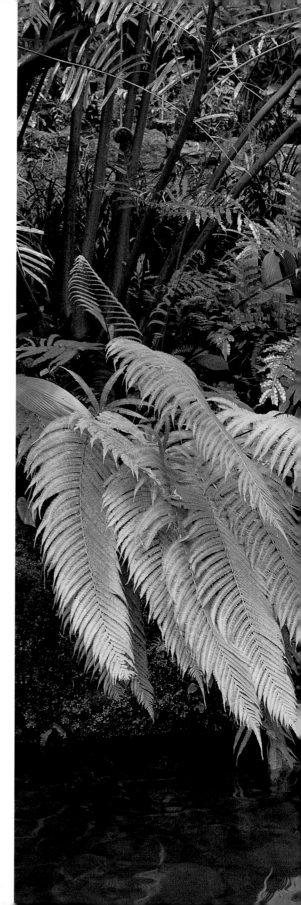

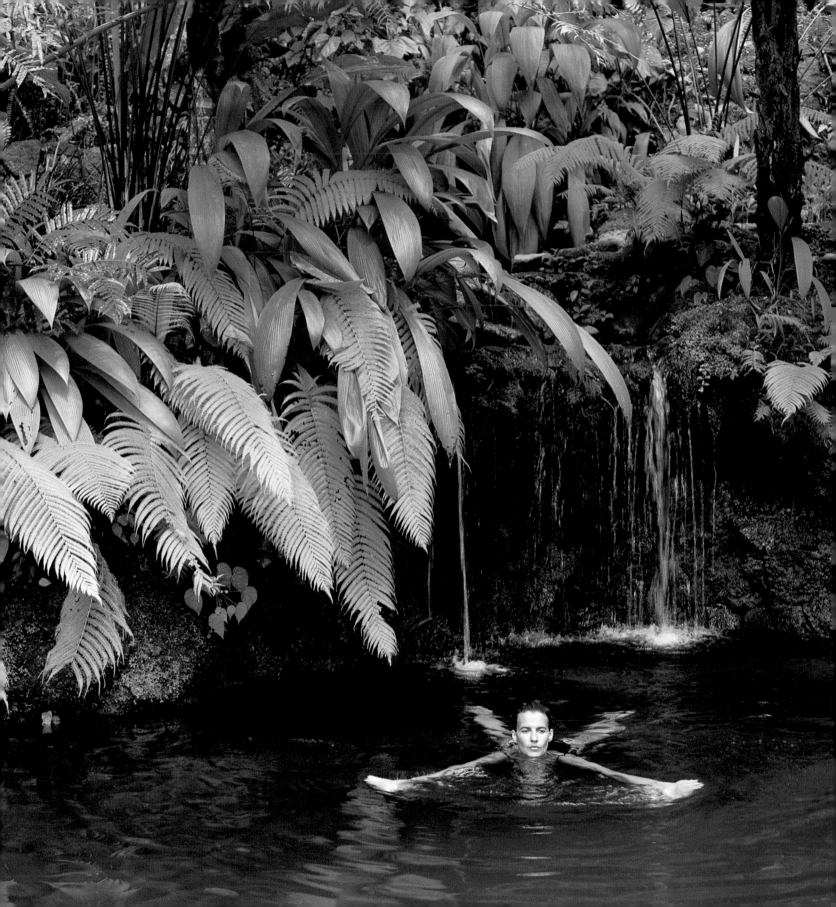

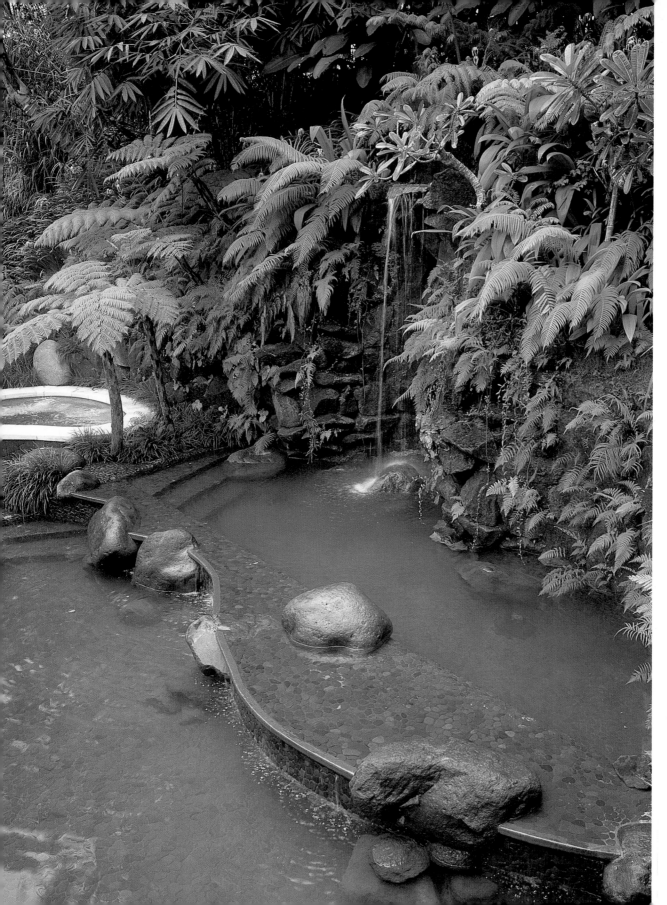

< The 'natural' spa experience at *Begawan Giri* (Wise Man's Mountain) takes visitors on a journey through terrain like this found at one of the villa's open-air bathrooms. The 25-acre estate is planted with 2,000 indigenous hardwoods and is filled with such flowering plants as heliconia, ginger and orchids.

> (*Clockwise from top left*) A hair perfuming treatment offered only at *Begawan Giri* literally smokes the hair with perfumed incense as it dries.

A jacuzzi at one of the villas.

The philosophy of *The Source* says that the more people are returned to nature for reflection, exercise and therapy, the easier it is for them to begin to experience their true inner healing and balancing energies.

Each of the five residences is drop-dead dramatic. They are testament to architectural achievement whereby built form and jungle fuse in super-statement. There is nowhere more stunning to stay – or recline for a massage – in Bali.

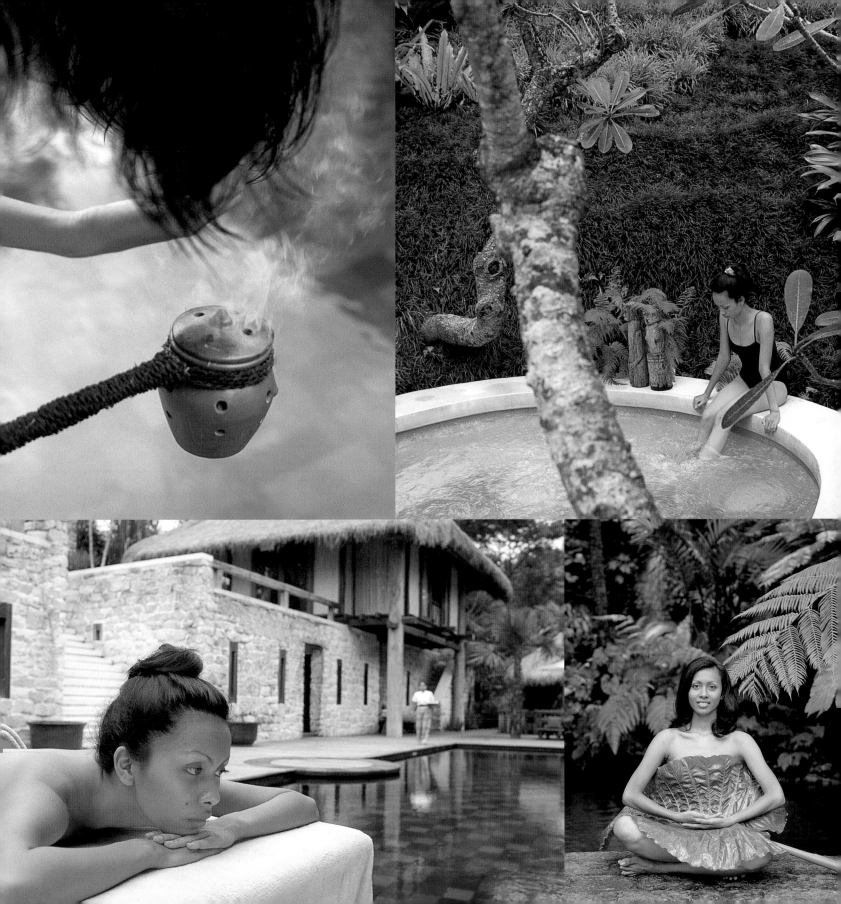

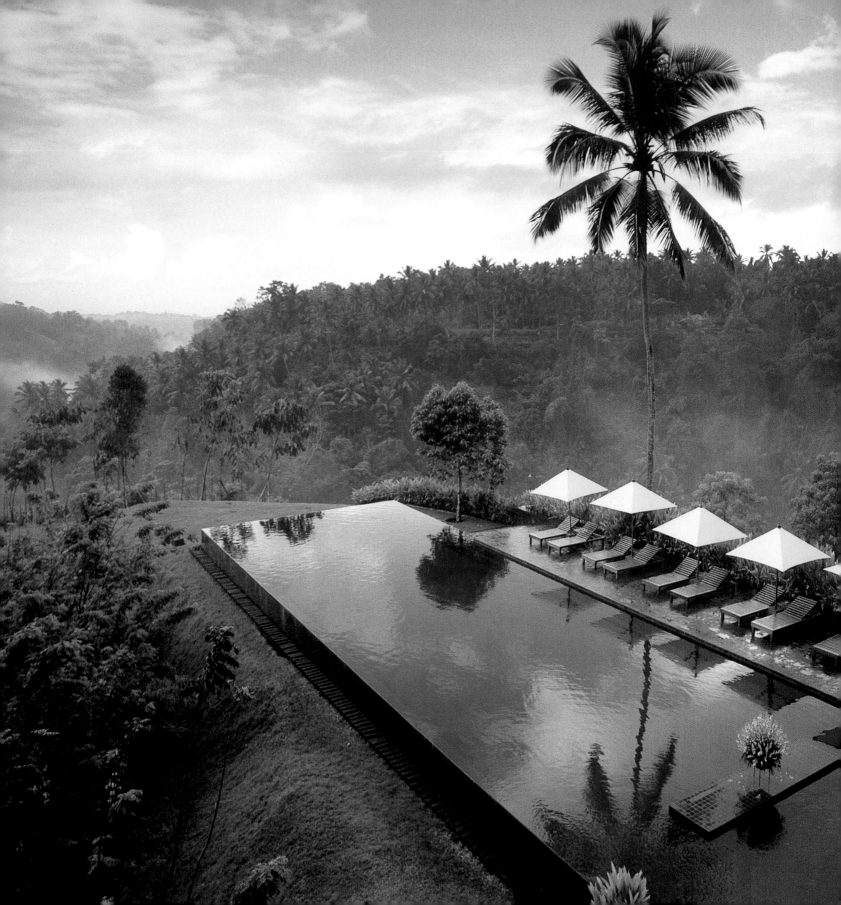

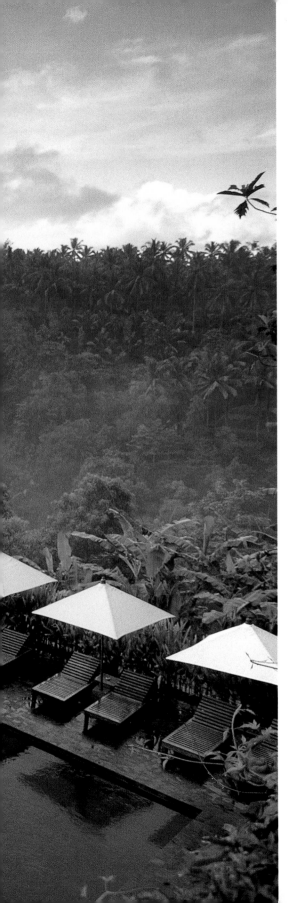

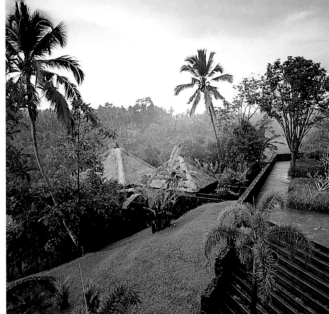

<< There cannot be many swimming pool spots in the world that take your breath away quite like this. A stunning slab of black water teeters on the brink of Bali's most dramatic river gorge. The silence here is almost busy with a sense of spiritual activity.

Mandara Spa at The Chedi

The sounds of lapping waves on Bali's coast are swapped for those of lowing cows and crickets in the hilly country of Ubud. Far from the madding beach crowds, nature remains raw and abundant up here and the spas adopt an earthy ambiance in tune with the powerful landscape surrounding them.

The much photoghraphed Ayung River gorge in Ubud is often cited as one of the most beautiful in the world and one of the many benefits of visiting the *Mandara Spa at The Chedi* is its dramatic setting on the lip of this valley, hundreds of feet above the river. The whole hotel, including the imposing infinity-edge swimming pool, seems to tumble into the sheer leafy jaws of the gorge, made soft by a landscape stepped with trees.

Even that nostalgic image of maidens bathing naked at the water's edge is realized by the local village girls. So just setting off for a spa treatment down a leafy pathway of moss-covered stones, kickstarts that back-to-nature feeling before you even disrobe.

This mood *au naturel* continues as you lie under a grass roof of cathedral-like proportions before an audience of big banana branches and flapping palms. Outdoor bathing diverges from the spa norm and takes on a whole new meaning: your bath is sunk into a loamy lotus pond twice the size of the double spa villa, making any presidential suite seem meagre by comparison.

The *pièce de résistance* here is the Mandara signature massage, an other-worldly combination of five massage techniques. It is rhythmically performed, like a dance over your body, by two therapists working together in synch. Book it.

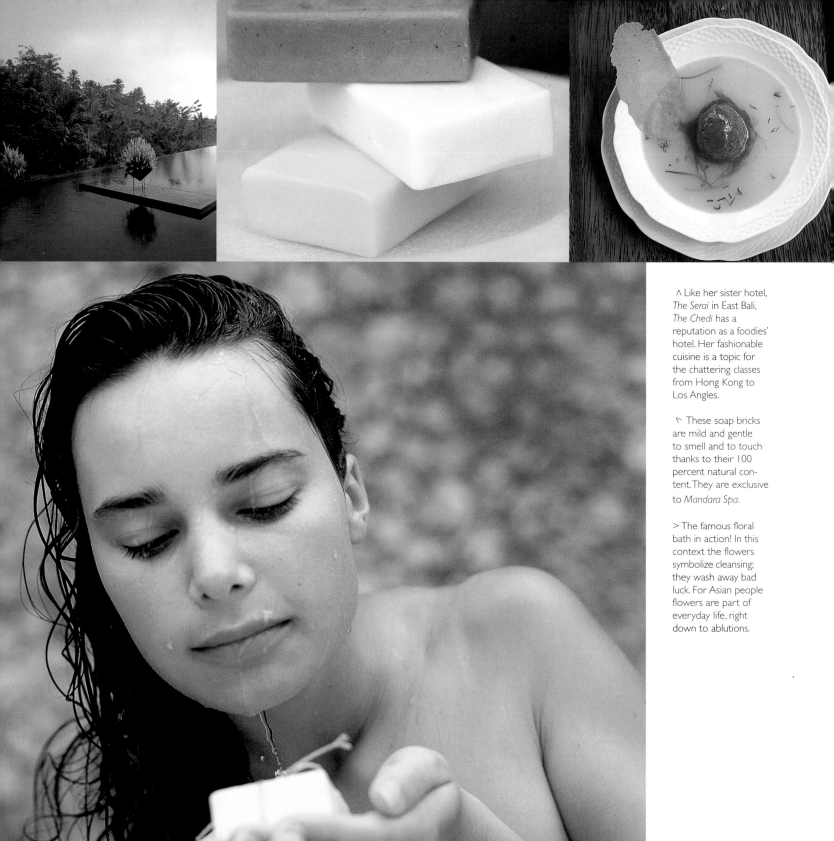

∧ Like her sister hotel, *The Serai* in East Bali, *The Chedi* has a reputation as a foodies' hotel. Her fashionable cuisine is a topic for the chattering classes from Hong Kong to Los Angles.

⌐ These soap bricks are mild and gentle to smell and to touch thanks to their 100 percent natural content. They are exclusive to *Mandara Spa*.

> The famous floral bath in action! In this context the flowers symbolize cleansing; they wash away bad luck. For Asian people flowers are part of everyday life, right down to ablutions.

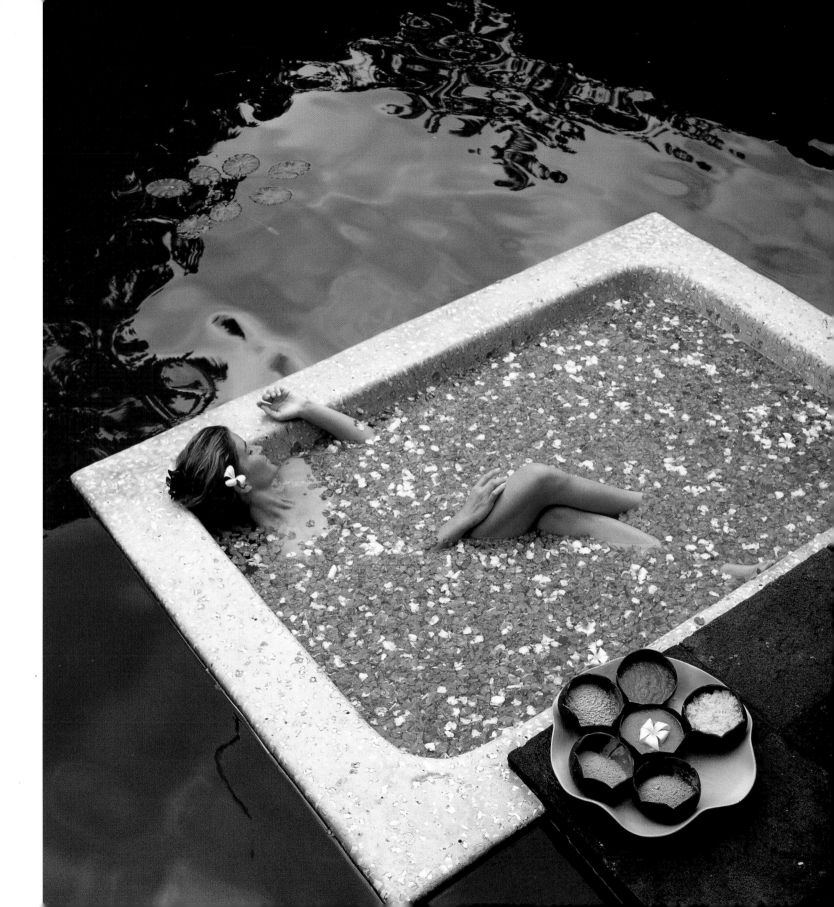

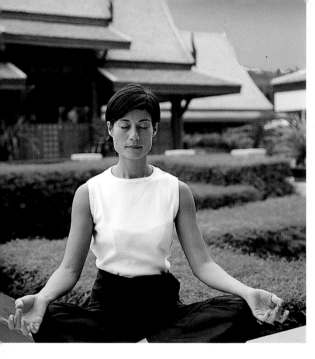

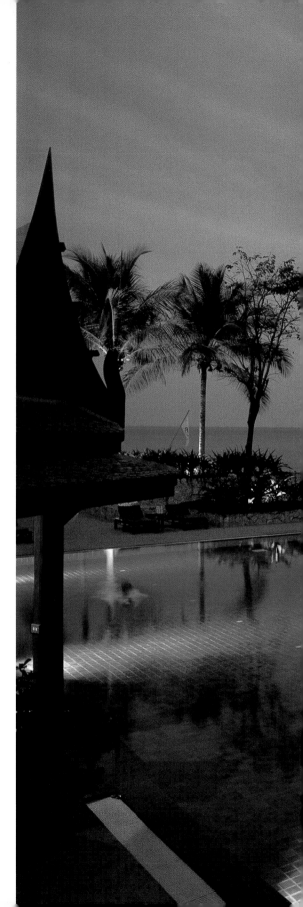

Chiva-Som

Chiva-Som is the only dedicated health resort that blends the quest for physical and mental well-being with exquisite luxury. Interwoven with the grace of the Thai people, this is a spa in a class of its own. As a result, the world of spa-goers can be divided simply between those who have stayed at *Chiva-Som* and those who have not. People cannot get enough of the kaleidoscope of facilities: scrubs, wraps and toning treatments, hydrotherapy in all forms, iridology and *Chiva-Som's* very own *equilibropathy*, medical guidance as well as meditation on the seashore. And this is only a sampling of what awaits guests at this visually sparse yet karmic resort.

Most people come for a period of between three and 14 days: these are spent blissfully in a bathrobe, yet busily pursuing *Chiva-Som's* 'mind, body, spirit' philosophy with a programme

tailor-made to help de-stress, overcome trauma or whatever. In between a session in the gym, an outdoor Thai massage and an introduction to *tai chi* at dusk, it's hard to find enough time to try the toys: water beds, flotation tanks, musical back massaging chairs…, let alone a gentle snooze by the pool.

Chiva-Som subscribes to the notion that diet and nutrition play a vital role in mind-body harmony. The kitchen caters for this with carefully controlled cuisine and a strict mealtime roster, offering a no-salt, no-fat buffet. However, the many lavish spa facilities and treatments take ones mind off food.

After all, at a US$26 billion 'haven of life' (the meaning of *Chiva-Som*) with a staff to guest ratio of four to one, it's hard not to subscribe to the maxim that health and happiness are one.

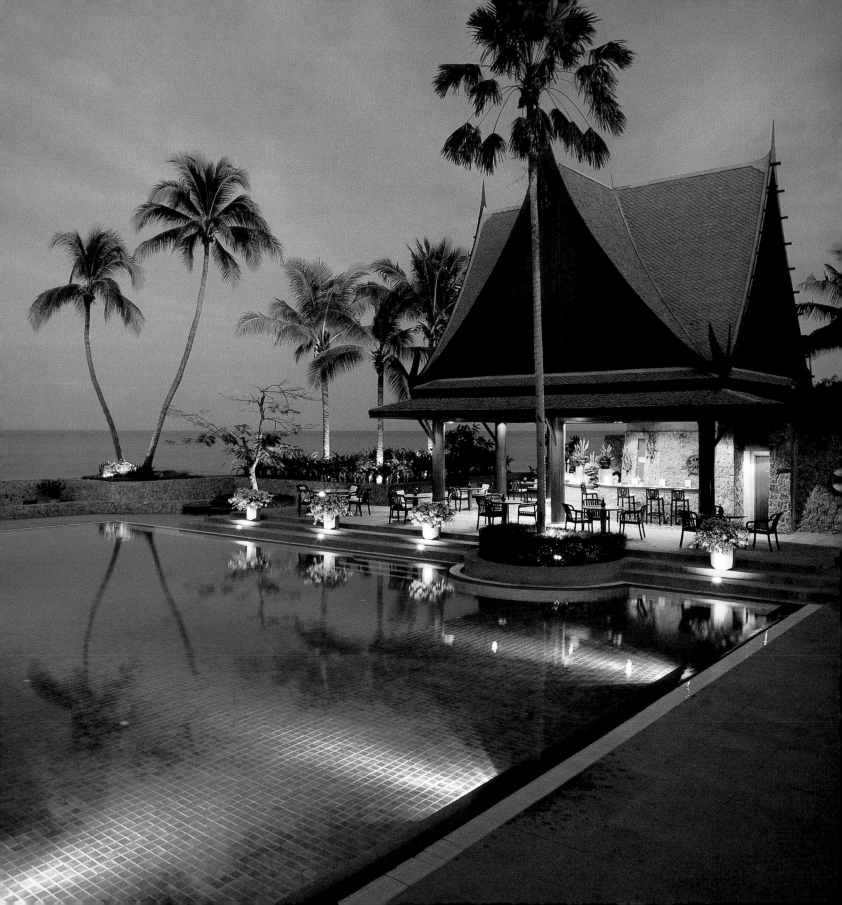

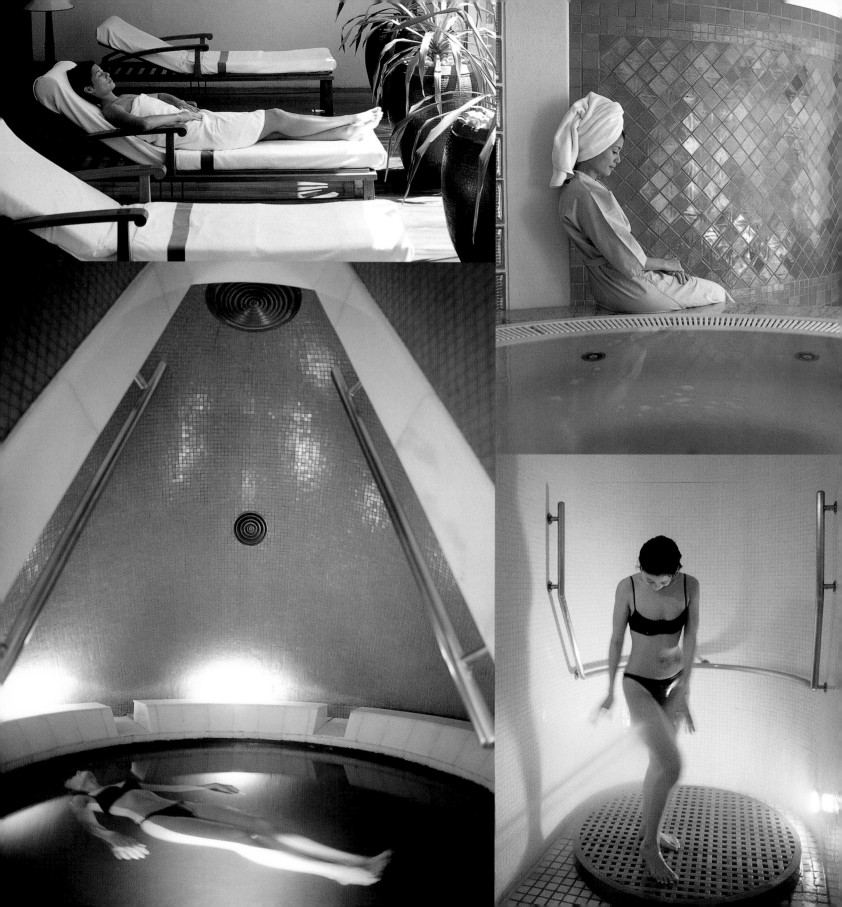

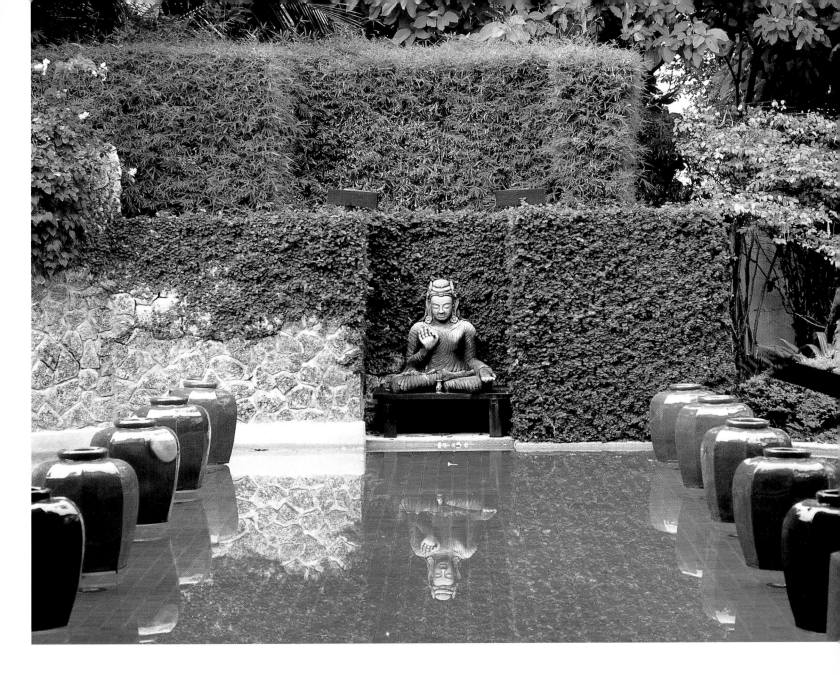

< The indoor spa area at *Chiva-Som* is enormous and full of facilities from a one-person jacuzzi pool to the innovative Body Blitz, a hydrotherapy treatment whereby high-pressure water jets directed at certain body areas work on lymph drainage to eliminate cellulite and smooth skin tissue.

<< Experts claim that half an hour in the Flotation Tank is the equivalent of eight hours' sleep. The temperature of the water mimics that of the body which is naturally supported by a saline solution. The feeling of suspension is designed to send you into limbo and leads to a deep feeling of inner relaxation.

∧ One of the inner courtyard views, in keeping with the pared down mood of the overall design style of the resort.

Mandara Spa at The Datai

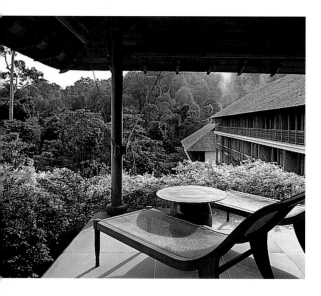

The Datai resort offers a 'tropical' spa experience in one of its purest forms – immersed in the jungle. Every sense is invaded while you lie, open to the elements, in one of the four spa suites that are mapped out along a wooded stream far away from the hotel rooms.

Try not to fall asleep to the rhythmic touch of your masseur. Cock open an eye and take in a full sweep of the surrounding rain forest. An open ear hears the chattering stream (whose sound is recorded on the hotel phone) and an open nose catches that pungent smell of rich, wet earth. With your third eye it's not hard to see a Dayak tribesman emerging from the trees to appear on the jetty of your spa suite. Stick to real vision and your visitor will likely be one of the many monkeys to whom this Malaysian slice of rain forest really belonged before The Datai arrived.

Aware of its intrusion into the precious equatorial forest, The Datai wears a mantle of sensitive design, somewhat like a hunting lodge, lying quietly under an ancient canopy in front of Malaysia's oldest rock formation from 550 million years ago.

The spa experience here, with its oriental massage and outdoor steam bath, enjoyed in the confines of a dark wood villa a hair's breadth from the fronds of the rain forest, is incomplete without a dawn nature walk. This gives the spa goer a clearer understanding of the greatness of the rain forest and how it affects us. Take for example the gatukola, a tiny ground creeper barely discernible among the thousands of species on Langkawi: apparently it is an aphrodisiac that reduces blood pressure and promotes long life while dilating the blood vessels and encouraging collagen production in the body. It is now pounded into face packs that we devour with relish in our quest for eternal youth! What better place to appreciate the harmony between health, beauty and the natural world.

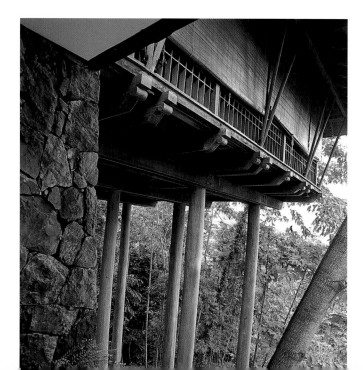

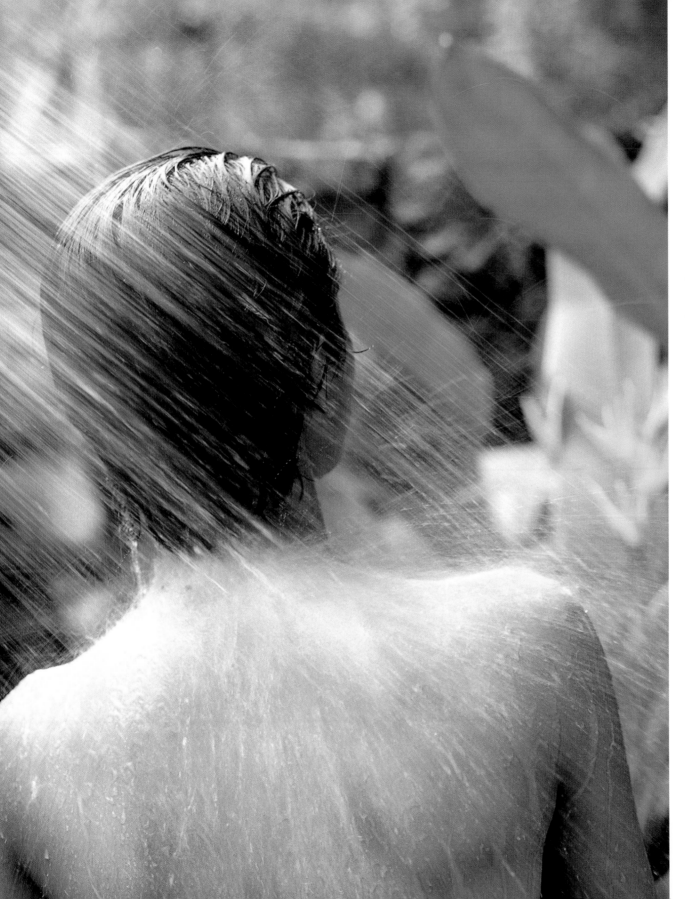

< The main body
of *The Datai* hotel,
Malaysia's first grand-
deluxe resort, is
almost 1,000 feet
above sea level. It
is enveloped by
centuries-old trees,
many with buttress
roots and jungle
twines, which
represent just a
handful of the 813
tree species found
on Langkawi, itself
an archipelago of 104
islands in the north-
west of the country.

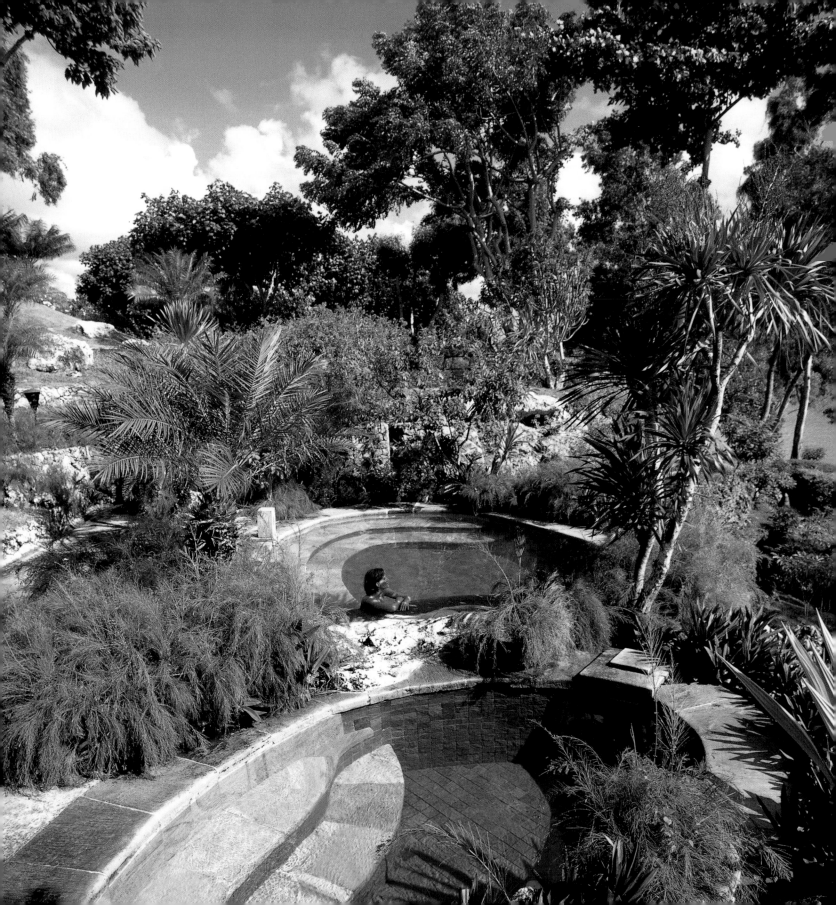

The Spa at Jimbaran,
Four Seasons Resort Bali at Jimbaran Bay

When it comes to luxury spa resorts, the *Four Seasons Resort Bali at Jimbaran Bay* has earned its stripes as one of the world's best, offering a seamless fusion between five-star amenities and local ambience. This same success has been carried over into the hotel's spa, also ranking as one of the best while maintaining its indigenous sense of the exotic: *gamelan* music, eastern aromas and a soul-soothing atmosphere where time has no role to play.

Unique to the *Spa at Jimbaran* is its Quiet Room: while painted in hot shades like the rest of the spa pavilion, it offers absorbing time-out as nurturing as the treatments themselves. Treatments here are high class and expertly devised in a menu that makes choosing almost as agonizing as the stress they aim to bust. The mere sound of a *Coconilla Scrub with Vanilla Beans and Coconut Milk*, a steamy 20 minutes in a *Peppermint and Lemon Grass Vapour*, or a *Wrap with Aloe Vera and Banana Leaves*, is a heaven-sent reminder that indeed this is the Island of the Gods.

Many treatments have been exclusively devised by Kim and Cary Collier, a couple who spent a number of years studying Indonesia's botanical heritage before launching their own spa consultancy. Their sensitive dedication to their work is reflected in the 'karma' that prevails among the therapists and hangs in the air. They also create the divine products used here. The texture, fragrance and ingredients of the spa's *Bali Santi* massage blend — coconut oil infused with essential oils of vetiver, basil and patchouli — speak for themselves. Sampling is believing!

While this spa is beautifully designed with indoor-outdoor treatment rooms offering that all-Asian frisson of showering naked next to nature, guests can be pampered in the privacy of their own residence too. These comprise walled courtyards, dining pavilion, bedroom, bathrooms inside and out and the famous private plunge pool and outsized tub. Indeed, some guests have been known not to emerge through their carved, painted, double Majapahit Palace front doors from arrival to check-out... and they have still enjoyed spa treatments most people only dream about.

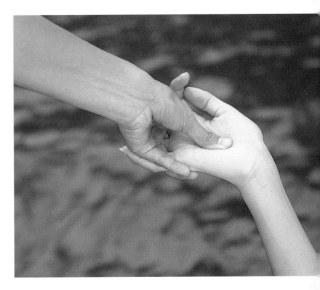

< The landscape design by Bali-phile Made Wijaya has won awards for this hotel. These hot and cold plunge pools reveal one of the many secluded spots found amongst the beautiful gardens. These took 500 labourers nine months of excavation and planting to create, according to what Wijaya calls his 'tropical Cotswold' aesthetic.

∧ Hand movements in traditional Balinese massage.

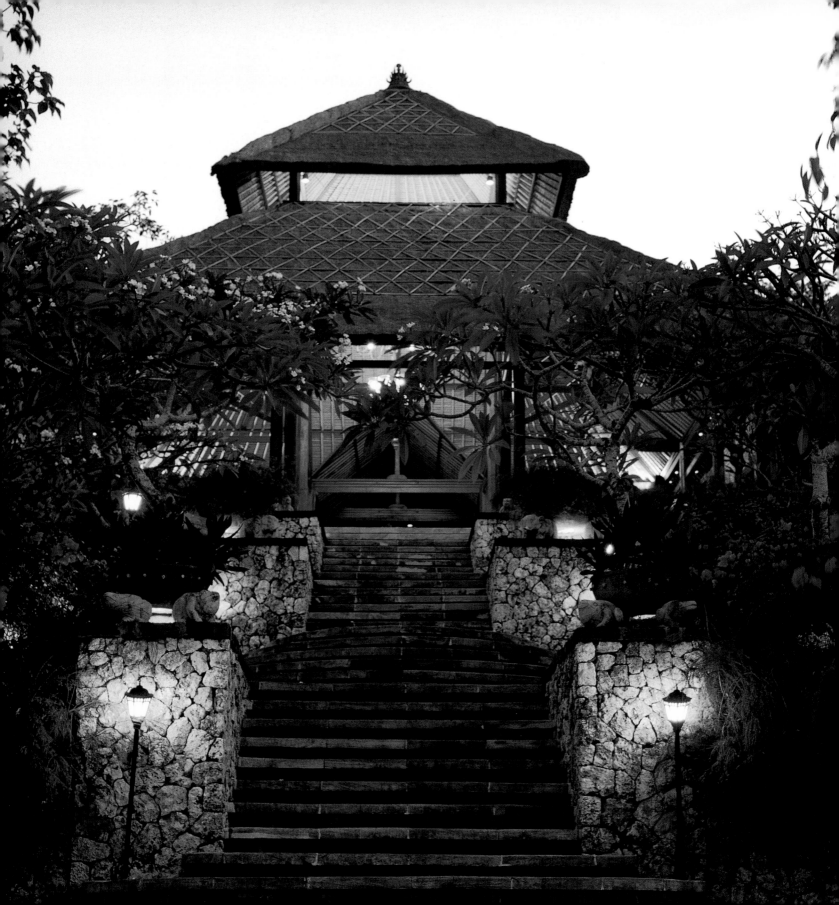

< A view up to the lobby from the main body of the hotel designed by Grounds Kent Architects according to a brief that combines the ambience of Balinese culture, namely a Balinese village layout, and the standards of a hotel in the 'World's Best' category.

> (Clockwise from top) This infinity edge pool is one of the resort's two public pools. However, this was one of Asia's first hotels to introduce private plunge pools in each of the villa suites.

All spa treatments are based on natural products rather than chemical preparations.

In oriental philosophy breath is synonymous with 'inspiration from the gods'. While normal breathing supposedly eliminates one third of toxins from our bodies, inhaling essential oils does more, stimulating our respiratory and nervous systems. This must explain why the scent from these oil burners enhances our sense of well being as soon as we enter this spa.

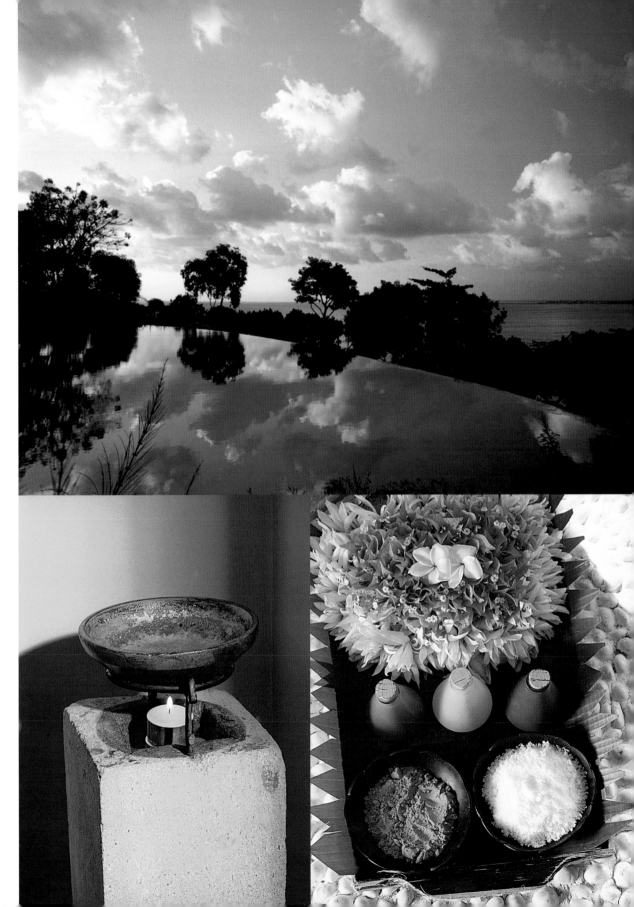

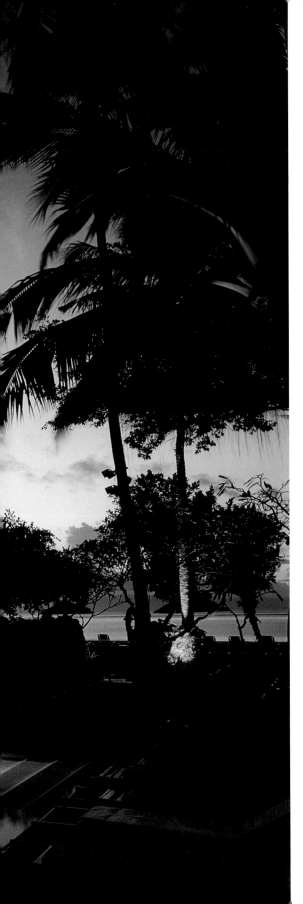

Spa at Bali Hyatt

Like so many Javanese words, *leha leha* says it all succinctly. It says peace, relaxation, day dreaming, an empty mind and lying prostrate gazing at the sky. In other words it says 'tropical spa experience', and more precisely the *Spa at Bali Hyatt*. This spa, designed and built as a Balinese village, is overhung with bougainvillea branches and lost in the midst of one of the most bountiful hotel gardens in Asia. It is *leha leha* at its most tangible.

In the raised, open reception of the spa, enjoy the honeyed taste of a health drink while you look at the stone maidens, hear the water that trickles from their pitchers, smell the flowers and touch the velvet pink of lotus blooms in the pond. Then walk through the Balinese doors into the inner sanctum for the ultimate *leha leha*.

The *Spa at Bali Hyatt* is special for the longer treatment programmes it offers. Once ensconced in your enormous private spa villa with sunken bath, shower and daybed outside and more within, it would be criminal not to linger for a two- or three-hour session. On top of this, the therapists here are blissfully slow at keeping time and quick at offering unexpected added extras: a floral foot soak at the start of every treatment, heated oil for scalp therapies, flower bowls fragrant with essential oils and an almost excessive change of fluffy towels. They even leave you with a fruit platter midway through your treatment for 20 minutes more of pure *leha leha* on your daybed. On leaving, it really is a case of pinching yourself back into the real world of signing the bill!

This spa mixes a complement of Asian-based scrubs, baths, masks and massages with Western jacuzzis, saunas, steam treatments and Australian essential oils. The belief is that its high-end customers like a tinge of familiarity to underpin the exotic.

< The *Bali Hyatt* was one of the first and remains one of the loveliest hotels on Sanur Beach. This swimming pool lies just back from the sand amid 36 acres of exquisite garden, designed by landscape architect Made Wijaya.

> The traditional Balinese village layout of the spa.

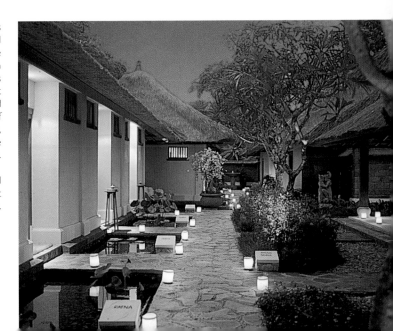

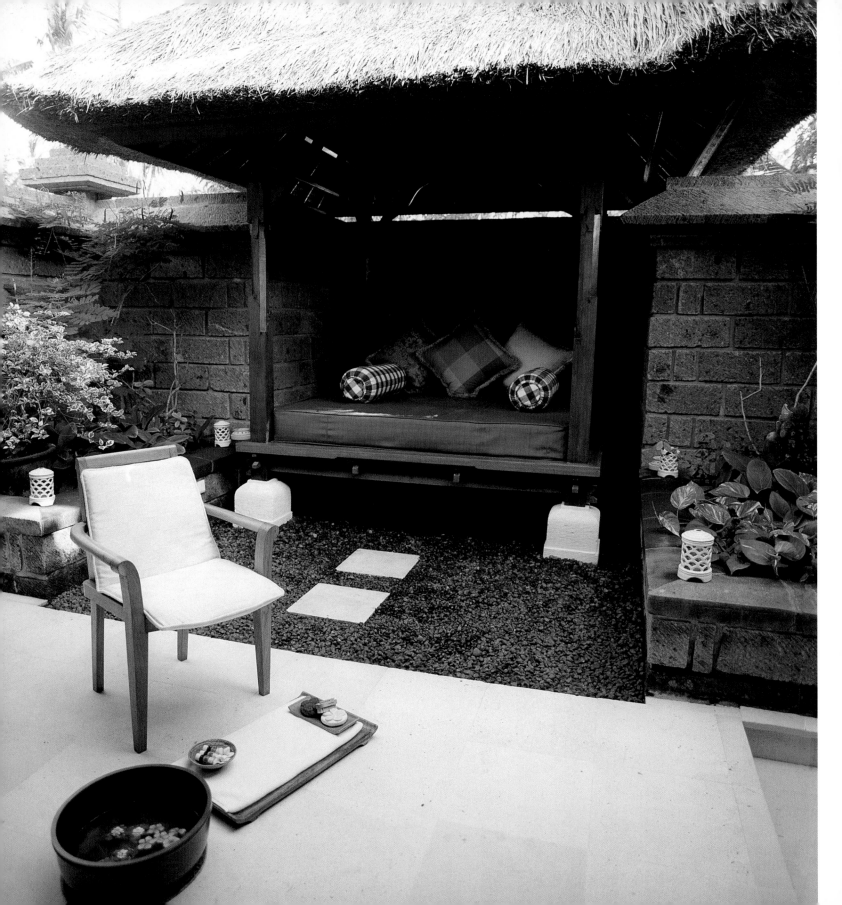

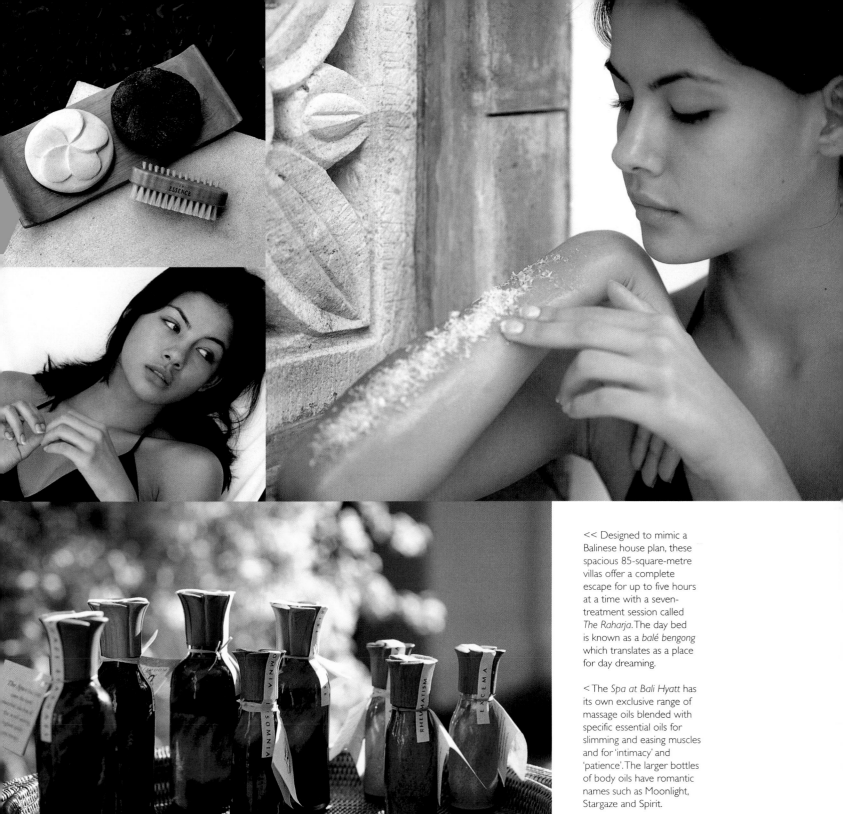

<< Designed to mimic a Balinese house plan, these spacious 85-square-metre villas offer a complete escape for up to five hours at a time with a seven-treatment session called *The Raharja*. The day bed is known as a *balé bengong* which translates as a place for day dreaming.

< The *Spa at Bali Hyatt* has its own exclusive range of massage oils blended with specific essential oils for slimming and easing muscles and for 'intimacy' and 'patience'. The larger bottles of body oils have romantic names such as Moonlight, Stargaze and Spirit.

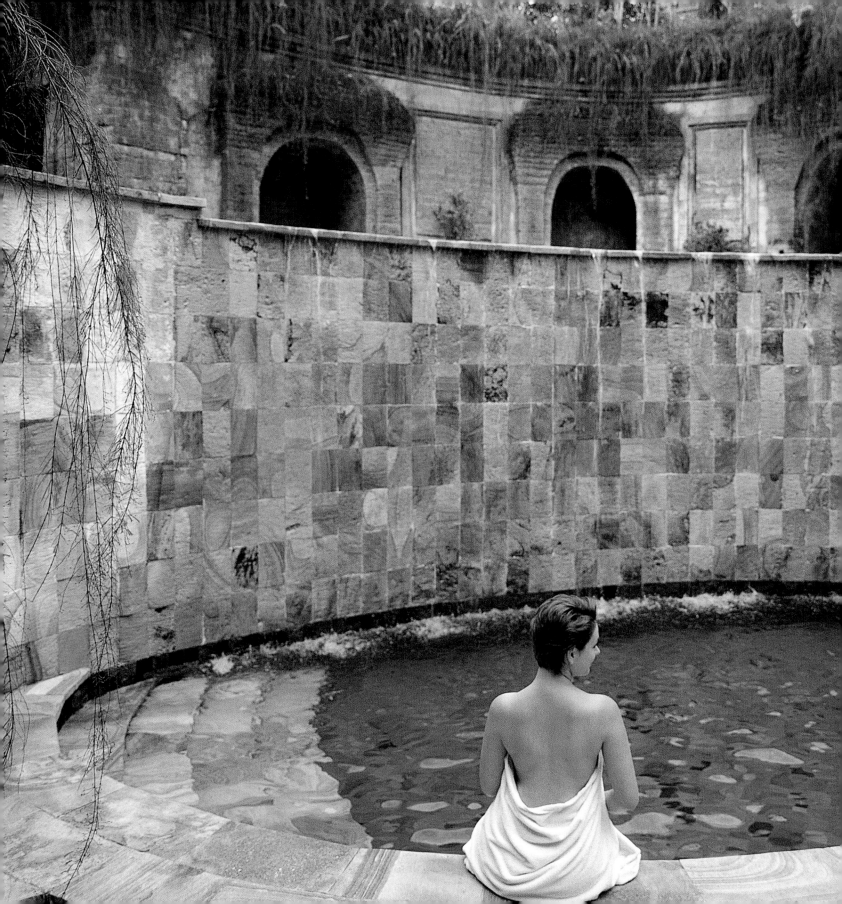

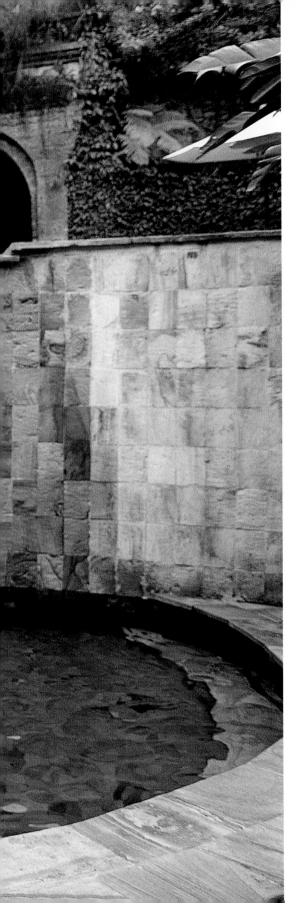

Mandara Spa at the Ibah

Somehow it is obvious – and all the better – when a hotel is family run, as in the case of the *Ibah*. In fact, it barely qualifies as a hotel with just eleven rooms, more akin to cottages each with its own distinct design.

The *Ibah*'s owners are an Ubud royal family who have held this dramatic site above the confluence of two rivers for generations. Like the proprietor's grandfather who would walk the one kilometre from the palace in Ubud to holiday and meditate on this spiritual slope, his descendant has sought to preserve it as an oasis of tranquillity for the lucky few who stay here.

"Staying at the *Ibah* is like being in love," says Tjokorda Raka Kerthyasa, its erudite and passionate owner, "you cannot explain it until you experience it." Somehow the light breeze, darting carp, murmuring water, nodding plants and sun-flecked stone seem to offer

a healing power that in no extent of the imagination can be anticipated.

This meditative mood remains unchanged in the spa, a panelled salon in the eaves, designed to cater for just one person or couple at a time, so as not to clutter its healing purpose. There's nothing clinical here. Instead, the dark teak wood and colonial furniture lend the spa salon a sense of decadence, accentuated by the massage boudoir, subtly lit behind tall curtains and lined with mirrors and stone deities that watch over you as you lie naked under their gaze.

Similarly, there is not even a whiff of the 20th century as you climb up the stone steps into your private jacuzzi overlooking the gardens below. This restful experience is best enjoyed at dusk when the *Ibah*, with its heavenly mantra, transforms into a galaxy of flickering oil lamps.

<>The owners of the *Ibah* refer to their hotel as a 'luxury homestay', although it is one of the most special on the Balinese spa resort circuit. It achieves, completely, the owners' dream to create a resting place for the senses, mind and heart.

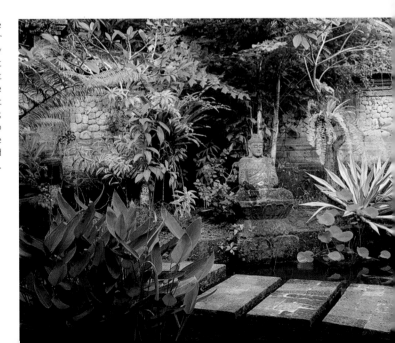

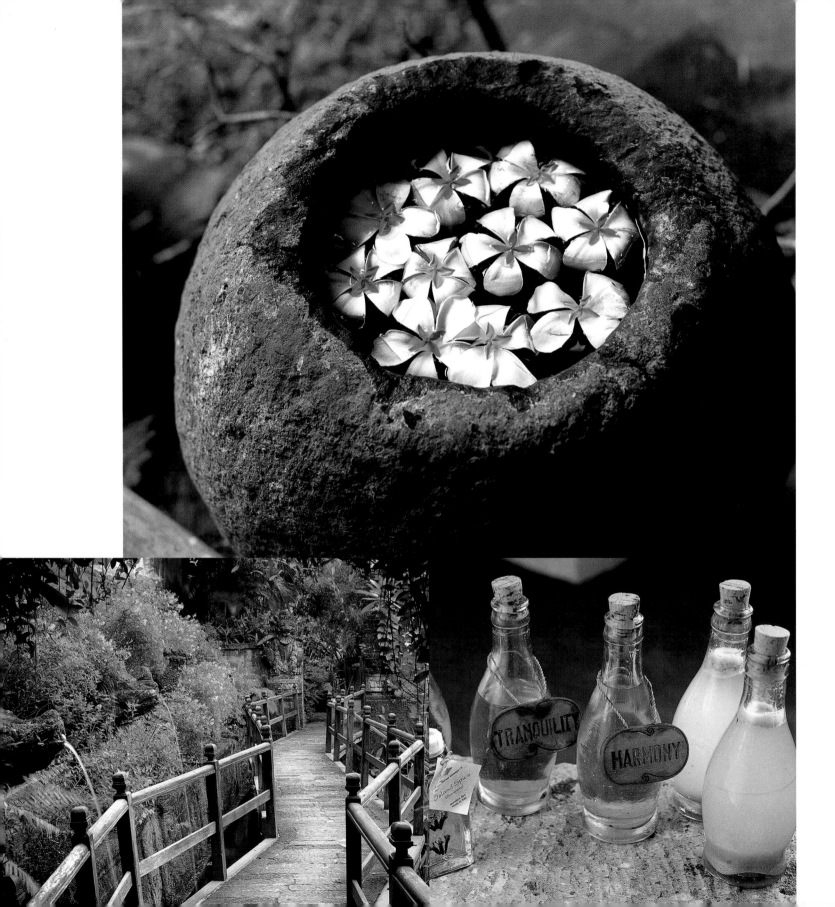

< The frangipani flower is the hotel's symbol. The blooms are arranged everywhere, in pots and to decorate statues, throughout the premises.

∨ The hotel is located in Tjampuhan which actually means 'where two rivers meet'. Balinese people believe that there is a flourish of *chi* (energy) at the junctions between two rivers which may help to explain why the spa experience at *Ibah* is such a meditative one. Bathing in a jacuzzi overlooking this vista is entirely memorable.

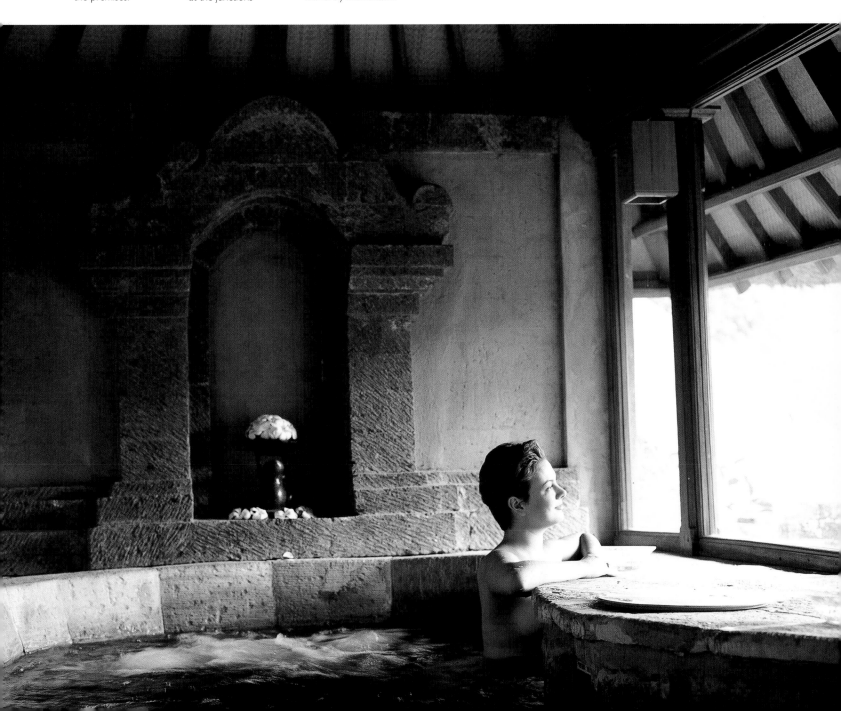

Nirwana Spa at Le Meridien Bali

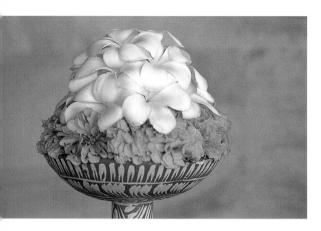

This spa is located in the shadows of Bali's venerated sea temple Tanah Lot and in keeping with the sacred role that water plays in our lives, it concentrates a large portion of its treatments on aqua-therapy. There is no more decadent place to immerse yourself in the beautifying and rejuvenating ritual of bathing than here amid the Balinese stone carvings that separate jacuzzi spots from plunge pools and outdoor showers.

The marine-style treatments follow the French favour for seaweed masks and wraps, including a hot algae rub-down, with their attendant claims for slimming and detoxifying. The one and a half hour *Tanah Lot Ocean* combination of massage, sea salt scrub and fragrant bath can be taken in an outdoor balé which overlooks the temple itself. This is perched on a little rocky islet off the beach with its own particular striking

aura whether delicately lit by the dawn sky or starkly outlined at twilight. The temple is linked to a 16th-century Majapahit priest who suggested to local villagers that this was a sacred spot.

The *Nirwana Spa* enjoys some of the spiritual peace emanating from Tanah Lot. Its airy reception looks out on an ornamental pool and further out over large, landscaped grounds. *Le Meridien* enjoys a far more tranquil location than the plethora of hotels just a few miles down the coast in the tourist stretch of Legian and Kuta. While the hotel is large, the spa is simple, clean and uncluttered, offering just the right send-off for the tropical scrubs, massages and water treatments it provides. More precisely, it has a relaxation room that really does its job, simply decorated and suspended over the pool to further add to the sublime ambience.

> A tropical spa treatment can be a spiritual awakening in itself. At *Nirwana Spa*, located in the shadows of one of Bali's most famous temples, the mood is further intensified. The setting, coupled with the ever-present sea breeze, is enough to send you so far away that it's hard to return to the real world.

↘ *Nirwana Spa* specializes in water and seaweed treatments, which have a strong purifying effect on mind and body.

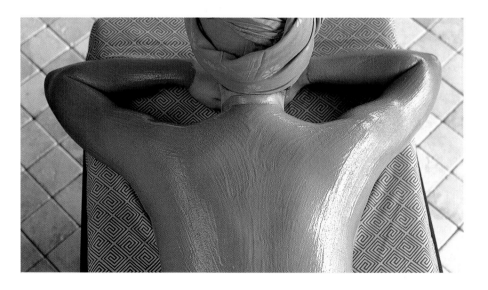

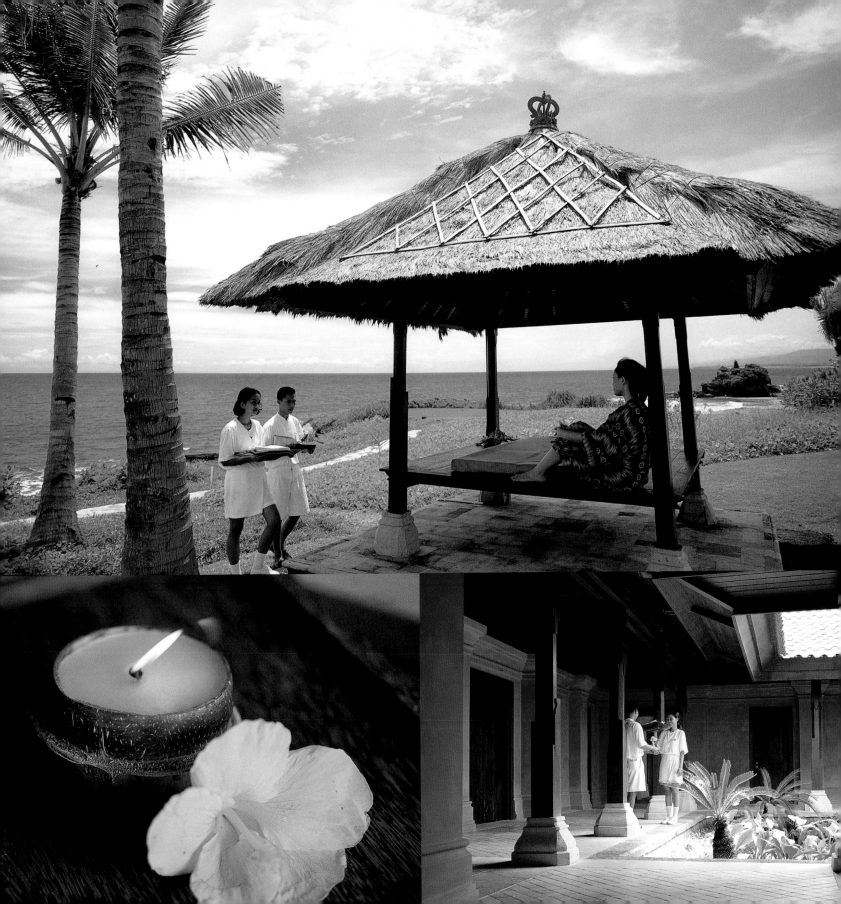

The Nusa Dua Spa

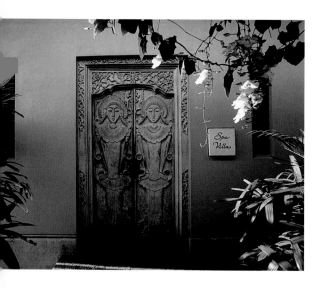

Water has historically been the key element in the traditional spa mix. This dates back to Roman times when over-indulgent sybarites travelled the land to take its curative powers by mouth or day-long soaking. Likewise, water is key to the Balinese way of life, ritualized in the form of holy water or *tirtha*. This, according to Hindu legend, is borne from the sea by a beautiful goddess and drunk by the gods for immortality. Water features strongly in most Balinese ceremonies when the people give thanks to the rains for making theirs an undisputed land of plenty, and to the sea as bountiful provider.

With these thoughts in mind, the spa at the *Nusa Dua Beach Hotel & Spa* was designed around water, literally as a series of pavilions encircling a lap pool. Banish visions of the sterile field of water found at fitness centres in favour of a skinny, turquoise tube overhung with flowering branches and underwired with a subaqueous sound system. Above water level, the sound of falling water that abounds adds to the languid mood.

Treatments focus strongly on Bali's natural medicine chest. Massages, rubs, baths, head, face and foot manipulation, and several indulgent combination programmes, have been devised by spa consultant Kim Collier. Collier has spent three years combing Indonesia in her effort to preserve the country's bottomless box of beauty traditions by offering them in a spa context. She has, in order to cater to global spa goers, blended some of her traditional findings with western techniques for some of the massages and facials offered here.

The *Nusa Dua* was Bali's pioneering Tropical Spa. It was opened in 1994, and has since been refurbished into a colourful complex where health and relaxation fuse under the palm trees.

> This is the largest spa in Bali with 26 therapists performing 80 treatments per day between them, yet it manages to retain an aura of calm thanks to the mesmerizing sound of pouring water and the heavy scent of tropical flowering plants.

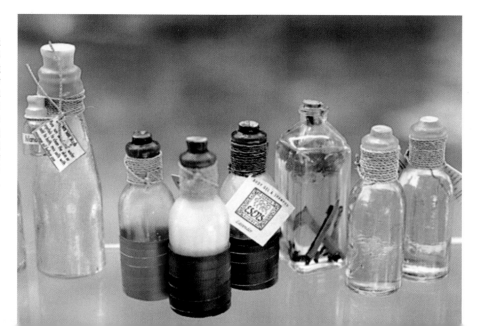

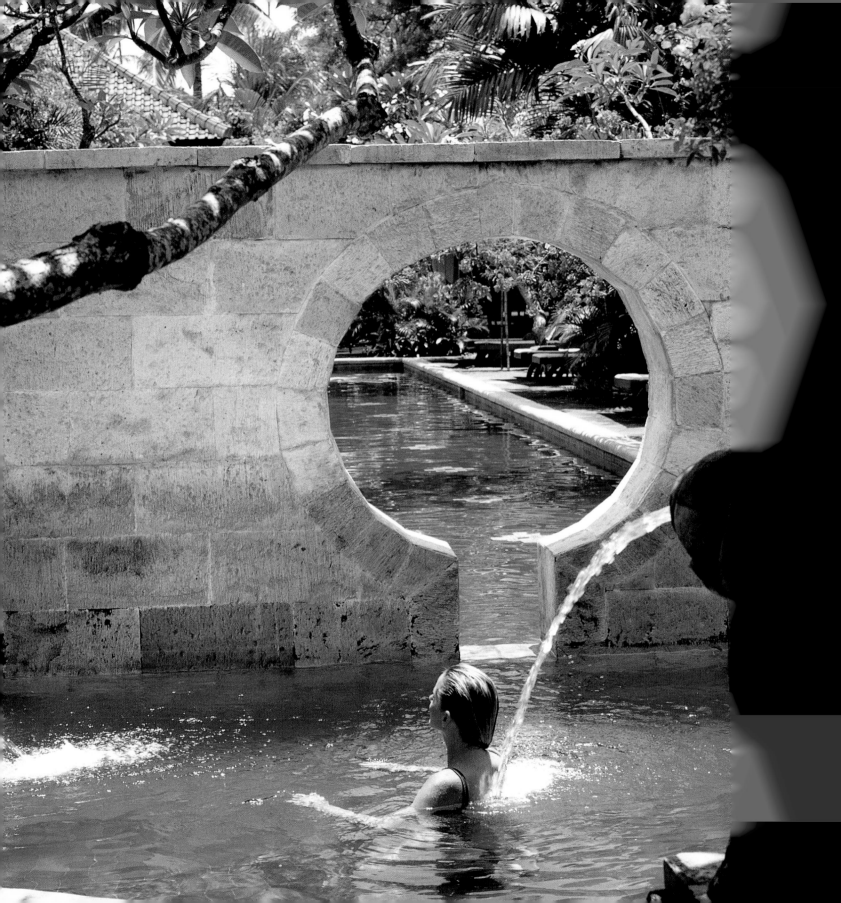

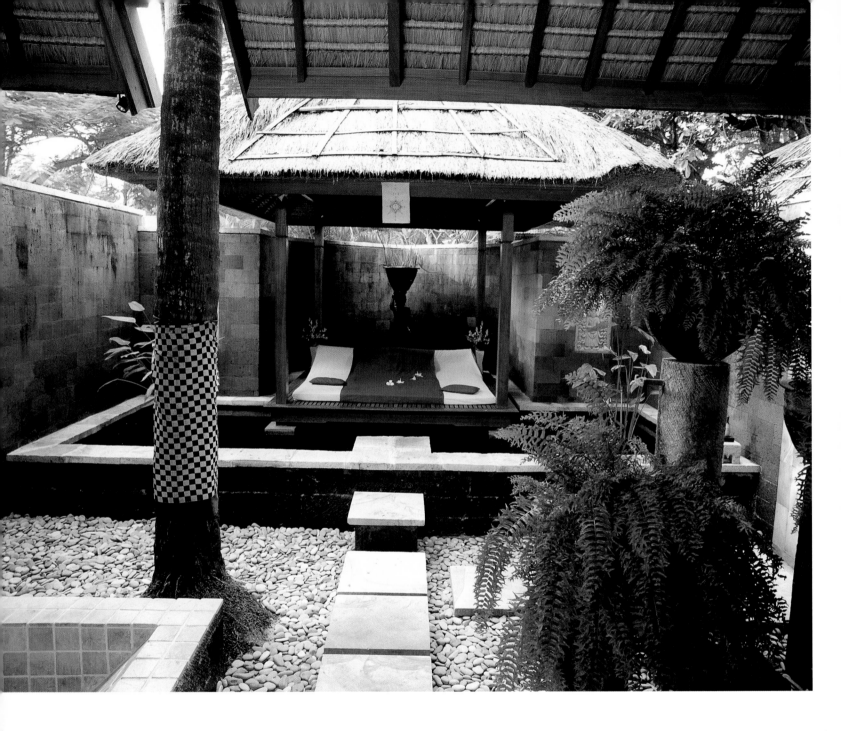

∧ One of the delights of a tropical spa is the outdoor treatment experience. This large and lavish outdoor pavilion is a secluded spot under a shady grass roof in its own walled compound.

>The *Nusa Dua Spa* is a puzzle of vivid Mediterranean colour. It is built as four pavilions linked by cloisters and shaded by the waxy blooms of the lampergia creeper.

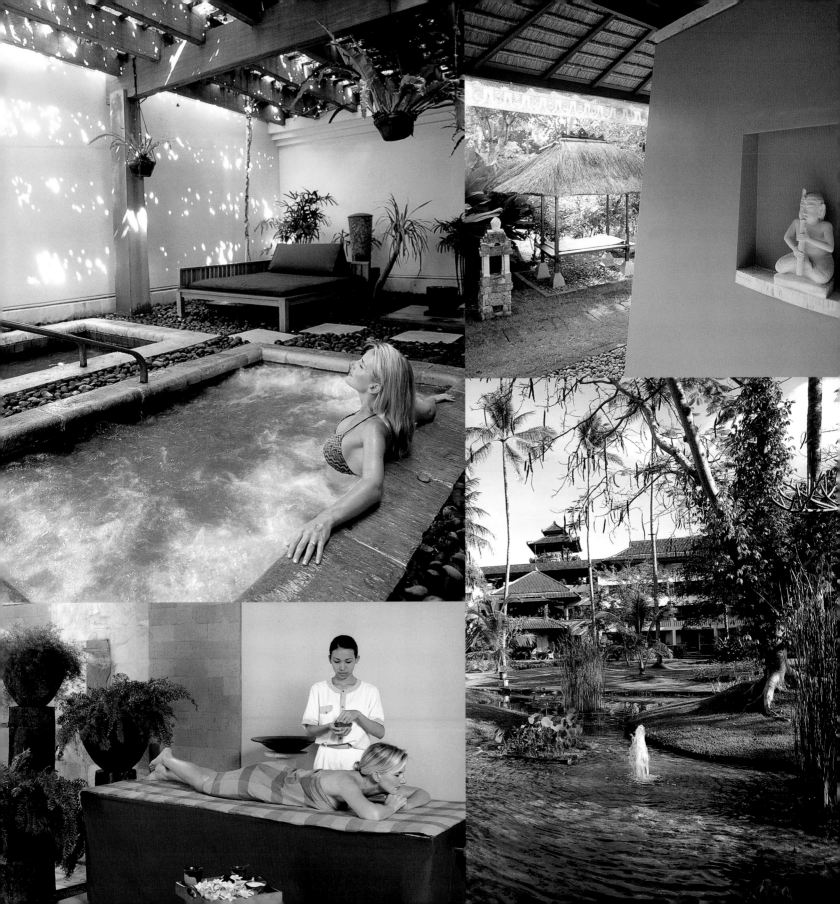

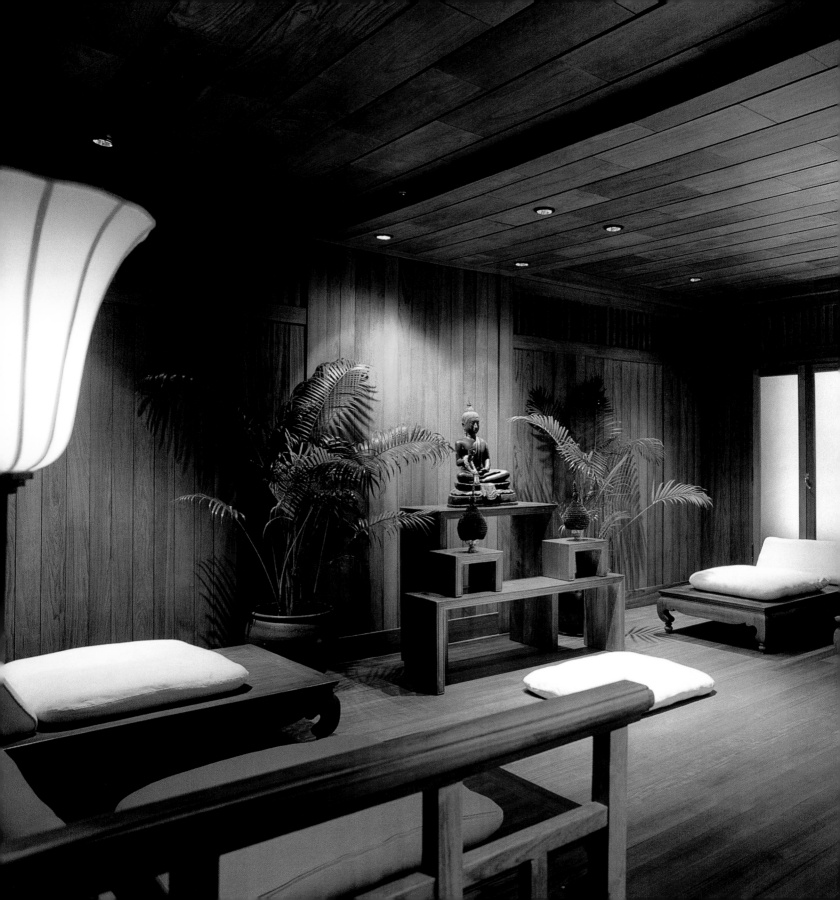

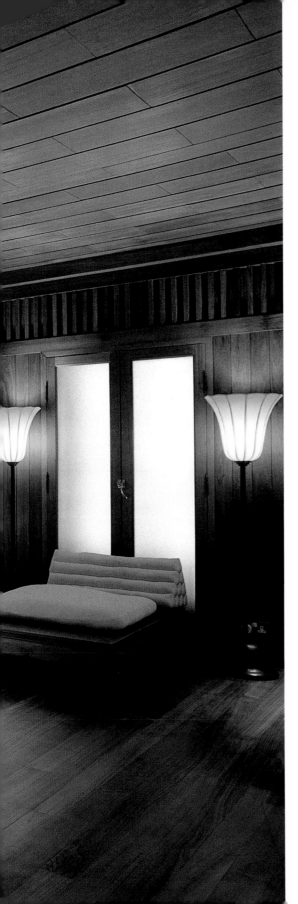

The Oriental Spa

A super-deluxe senior among Asia's spas (the oldest in Thailand just five years after opening), *The Oriental Spa* remains long on sophistication and short on pretension (new massage beds are still in storage because in reality a mattress on the floor is fine). Tucked away in a colonial-style house, the spa is cocooned in golden teak-wood with no unnecessary features and no communal area to cheapen the experience. Here is a city retreat where serenity reigns.

In the privacy of your own spa suite, high ceilings emphasize that this is, indeed, a temple of well-being. The simple, white mattress indicates that this is traditional Thailand and a family-sized shower, which spurts in all directions, reminds us of this spa's high-tech attention to detail.

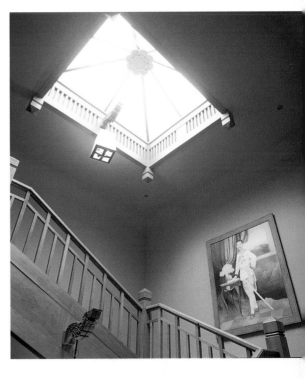

The treatments themselves have, over recent years, reached the lips of the chattering classes, presidents and princes, such is their exotic and effective nature. Papaya, mud, honey and herbs take their traditional places next to international favourites and one-off remedies such as *Jet Lag Massage* (a combination of Swedish and Thai techniques that releases energy). For all of this, the Thai therapists, living as Buddhists in the urban tumult of Bangkok, understand the nature of tranquillity.

The Oriental Spa is part of *The Oriental*, the legendary Asian hostelry that has hosted such world-famous authors as Somerset Maugham, Graham Greene, Noel Coward and Joseph Conrad who originally stayed there as a marine officer awaiting his first ship as captain. It is a hotel that has been synonymous with style for much of its 120-year history and is deemed by many as the finest hotel in the world. Its spa, reached by boat across the river from the main buildings, deserves a similar accolade.

< Despite being in the heart of Bangkok, *The Oriental Spa* offers one of the best antidotes to executive burnout. Start the relaxing process in this meditation room which, like the rest of the spa, is panelled in Thailand's golden teakwood chosen for its rich patina.

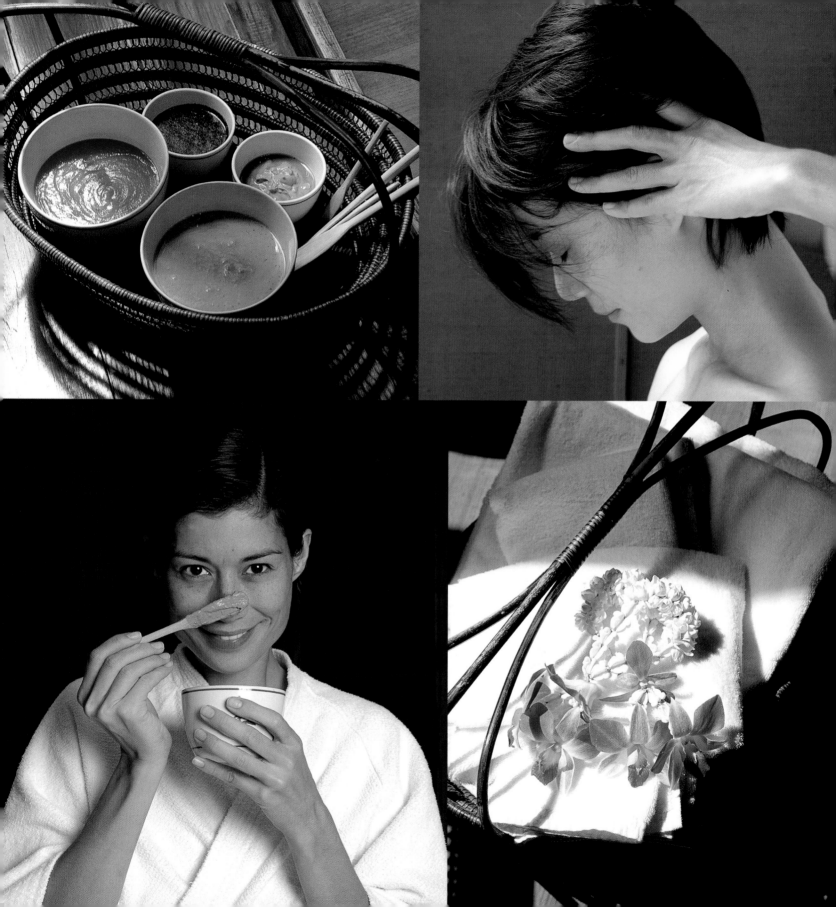

<< Ingredients for traditional Thai body treatments look and smell good enough to eat. These recipes contain sesame oil and seeds, milk, honey and various herbs.

< The head is a key zone in Thai massage therapy. Pressure along the scalp lines can increase blood flow to the head as many of the body's nerves congregate here.

The Oriental Spa offers an exclusive head massage for those who are pregnant or feeling a little delicate in the stomach.

V The Spa reception.

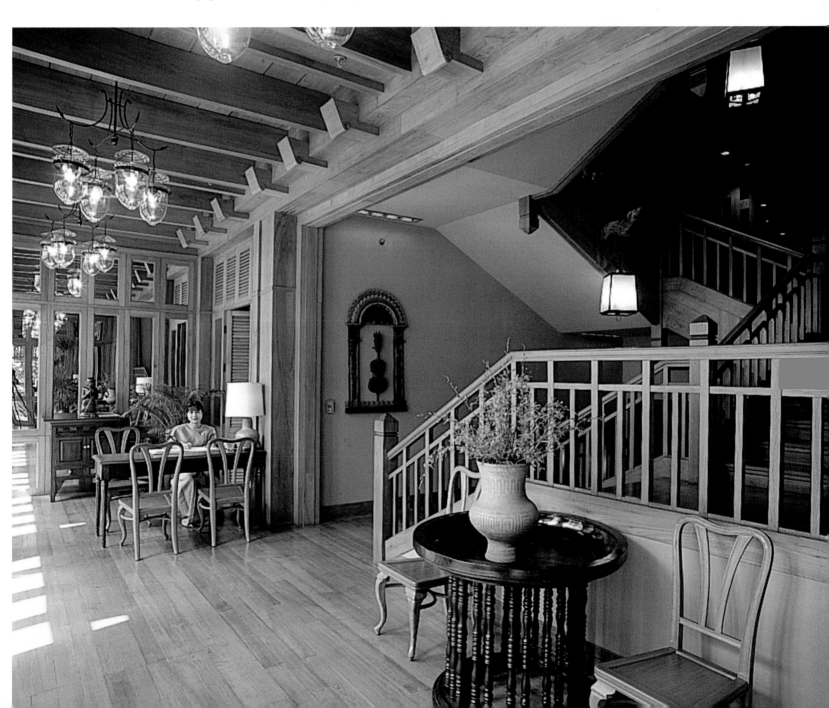

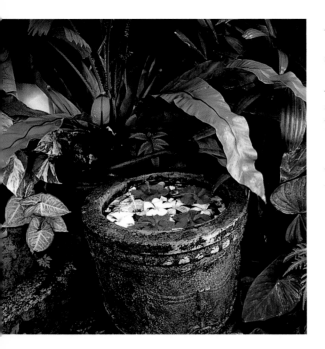

The Pita Maha Private Villa Spa

A session in the *Pita Maha Private Villa Spa* makes you feel like the royalty that actually owns it. You may even be lucky enough to have the luxury spa villa – a three-tiered, herbaceous hangout – all to yourself (and partner), giving you the opportunity to plunge naked into the hot and cold whirlpools, the swimming pool and the spring water flower bath at your whim. Each of these pools sidle up to a steep precipice overhanging the prodigiously beautiful Oos river valley, so that you are bathing on what seems like the edge of the world, while still in a veritable tropical paradise.

The 400-square-metre spa villa complex is inundated with waxy leaves that reach out to tickle you and a garrulous chorus of frogs that croaks into song at dusk. While there is only a small diet of seven traditional-style scrubs and massages, this is much more of a sanctuary than many of the island's larger and supposedly plusher spas where you are herded in and out according to a strict treatment roster. What the *Pita Maha Private Villa Spa* lacks in resort-style veneer (no pizza head showers here), it more than makes up for in charm and tranquillity. The sauna and steam rooms are hewn from the rock face, the outdoor shower's soap dish is a tree trunk and the herbal refreshers are poured out of a teapot carved from a coconut shell.

All of this happens in a charming hotel on the outskirts of Ubud. It is as far away in spirit as it is possible to get just three minutes from one of Bali's major tourist towns. Owned by a local prince, *Pita Maha* boasts a standard of workmanship found only in Balinese palaces. Its rooms, laid out like a village compound with their own private pool, are as large as a good-sized apartment.

> The medley of pools adjoining the private villa spa is set into the hillside, overhanging the Oos river valley which faces the rising sun; *Pita Maha* translates as the "Great Shining".

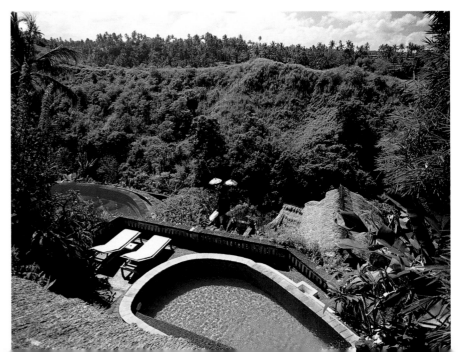

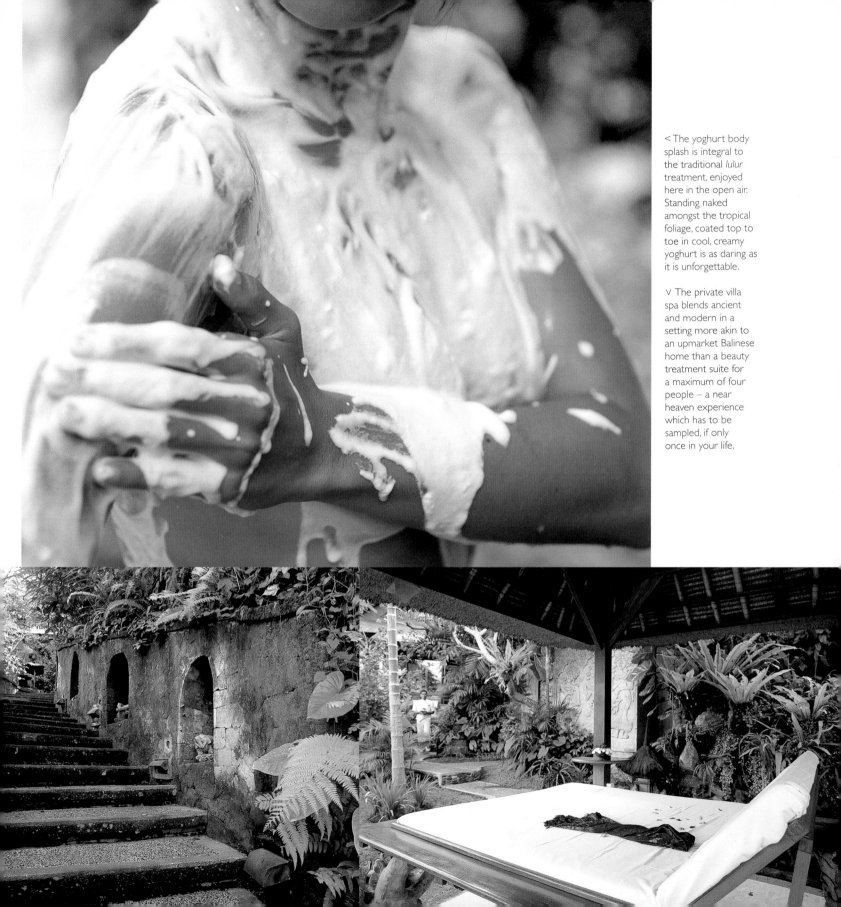

< The yoghurt body splash is integral to the traditional *lulur* treatment, enjoyed here in the open air. Standing naked amongst the tropical foliage, coated top to toe in cool, creamy yoghurt is as daring as it is unforgettable.

∨ The private villa spa blends ancient and modern in a setting more akin to an upmarket Balinese home than a beauty treatment suite for a maximum of four people – a near heaven experience which has to be sampled, if only once in your life.

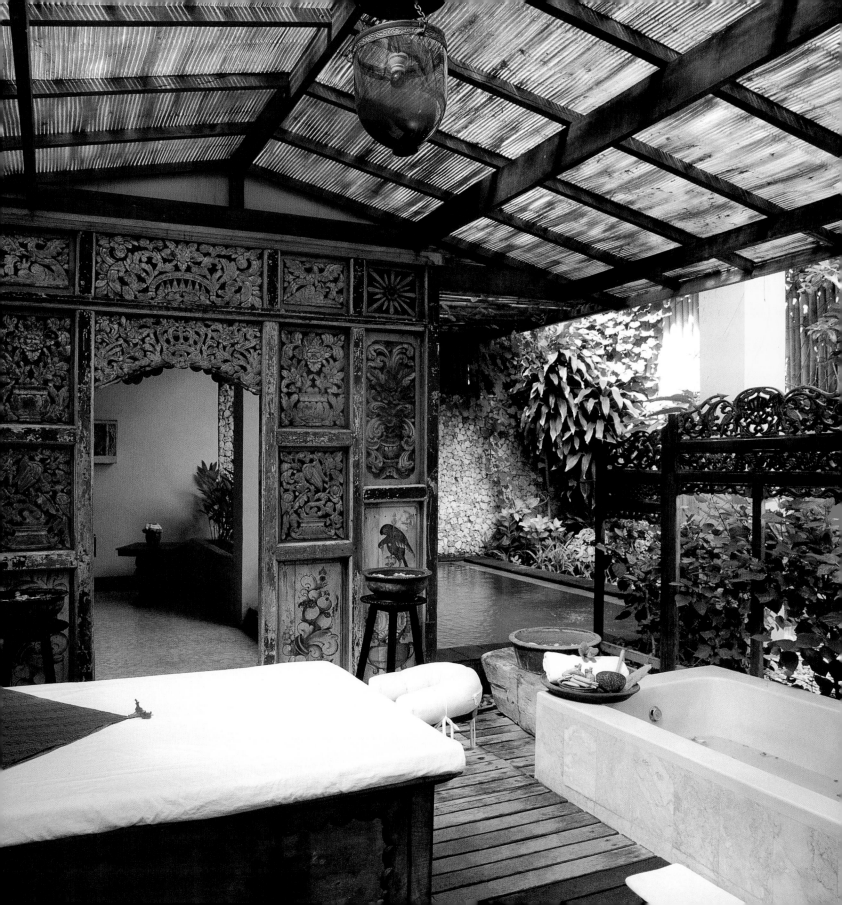

Spa at Hotel Tugu

Traditional is an over-used word in Balinese spa speak, but none can make the claim as faithfully as the *Spa at Hotel Tugu*. Here, if it weren't for the chrome taps, the treatments areas would unannily replicate colonial times, right down to the 100-year-old massage beds, wrought-iron barber's chairs and carved and painted wooden mirrors where the glass has gone fuzzy at the corners.

The decor of the three spa treatment areas, scattered among ten thatched sleeping pavilions, falls neatly in line with the rest of this 26-suite hotel. Put simply, it tells the story of several hundred years of Indonesian culture. It could be described as a 'museum boutique hotel' honouring its owner's passion for history. He built it in a solitary landscape behind the beach at Canggu to house the overflow of his own personal collection of antiques.

In the same way, spa treatments here have veered little from those therapies practised centuries ago. There are no manufactured products here; a large fruit platter displays most of the

body scrub and facial ingredients, bubbly glass bottles contain the massage oils made in Java: avocado, jasmine, *sukira* and coconut. Bowls of kitchen cosmetics bear testimony to old-style beauty routines such as honey for face lifting, burnt rice stalks to treat grey hair, yoghurt for washing, and raw eggs and candlenuts for other treatments.

The mood of yesteryear inspires the imagination and treatments somehow feel better in a truly authentic setting. The owner's wife, Dr Wedja Julianti, has personally devised the treatment menu and she concocts bespoke herbal potions for guests' ailments. This all adds to the home from home charm that *Hotel Tugu* has captured.

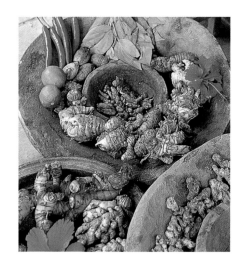

< The *Molek Seger Waras* (meaning "fresh, light and healthy") is fitted with antique Javanese room dividers and 100-year-old massage beds which are hollow inside to safeguard valuable belongings.

⁊ A selection of roots and rhizomes used in the preparation of traditional treatments.

> The dentist's chair is one of the many old pieces of furniture which adorn this unusual hotel.

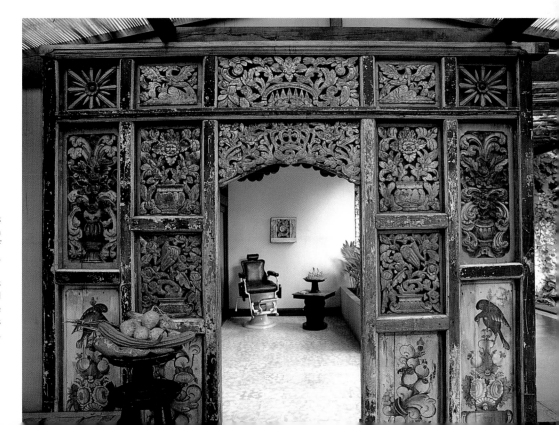

∨ All ingredients used here are natural.

> The *Kamar Solek* is translated as a room where a Javanese lady worked on her beauty regime in times past.

This 200-year-old wooden structure, used today for scalp and facial sessions, was once the outer part of a bed of the king's minister in Sumenep in East Java.

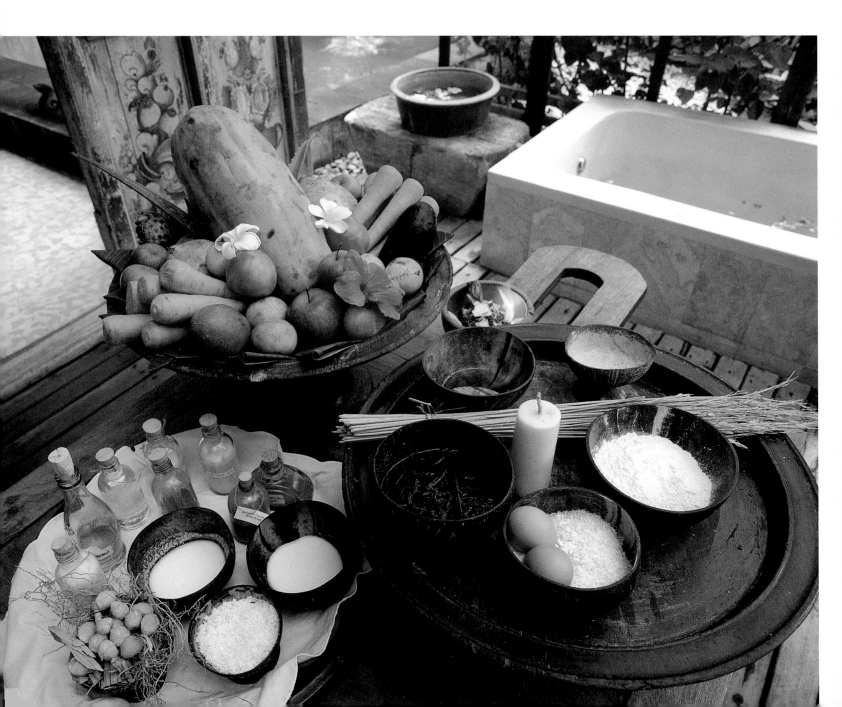

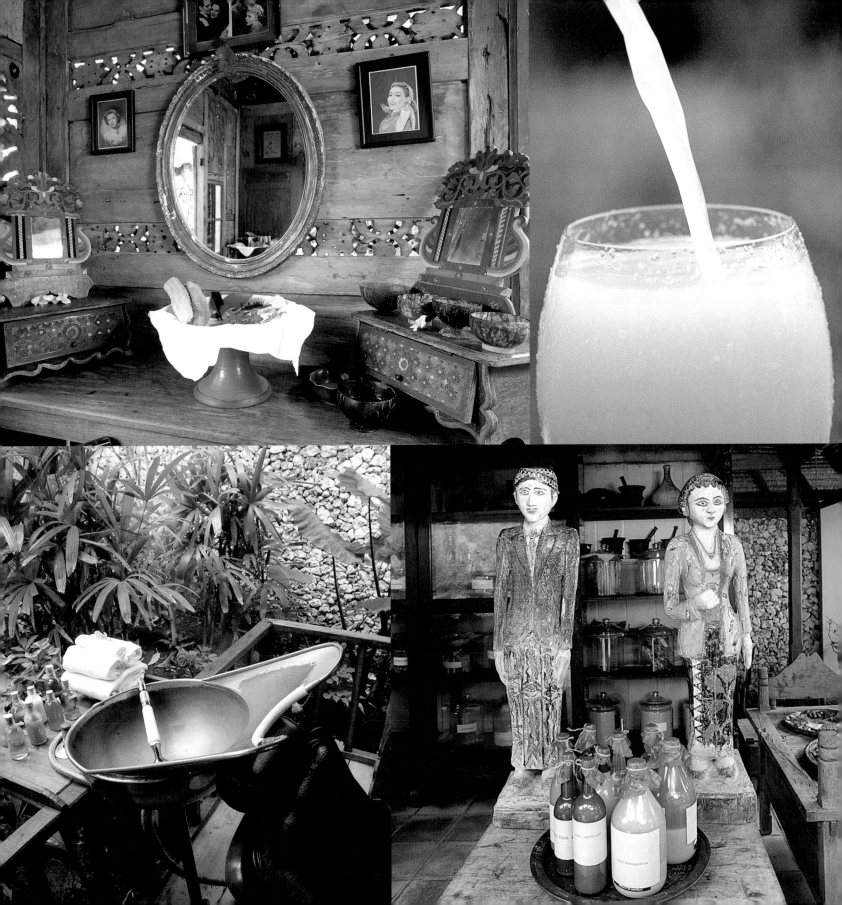

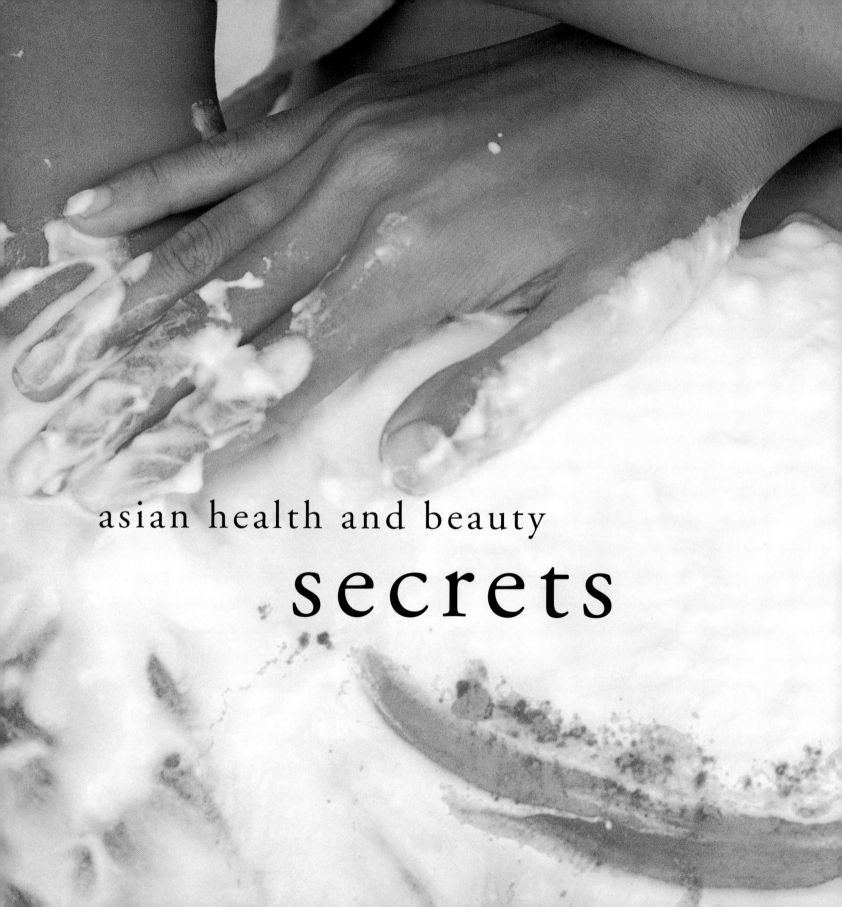

asian health and beauty
secrets

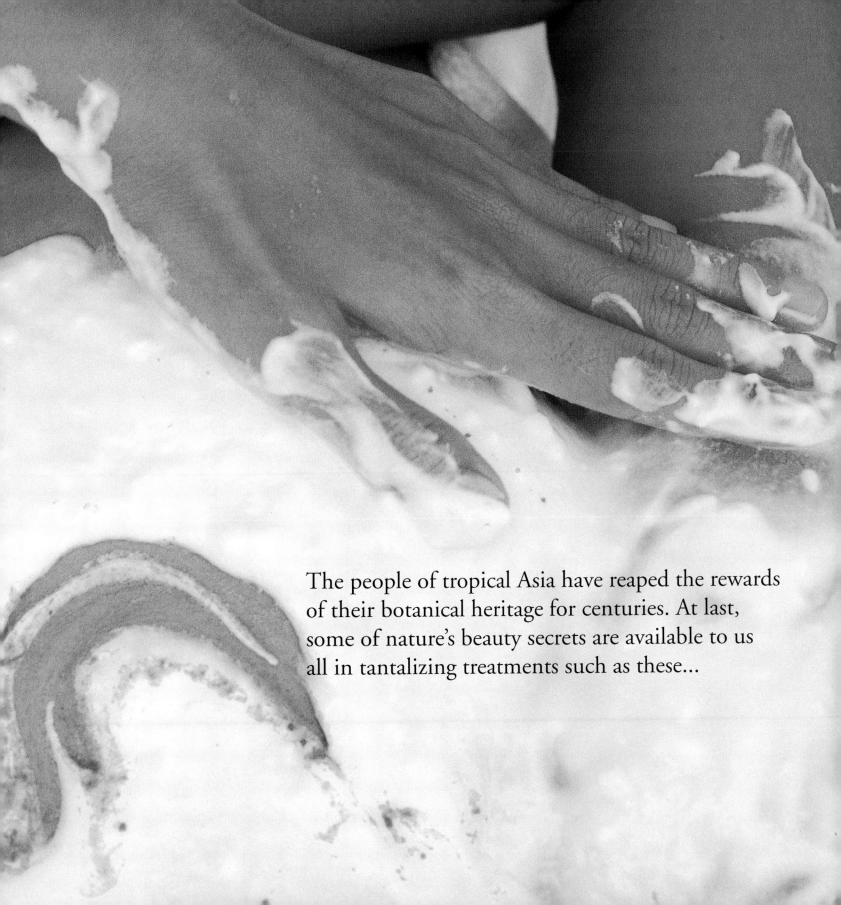

The people of tropical Asia have reaped the rewards of their botanical heritage for centuries. At last, some of nature's beauty secrets are available to us all in tantalizing treatments such as these...

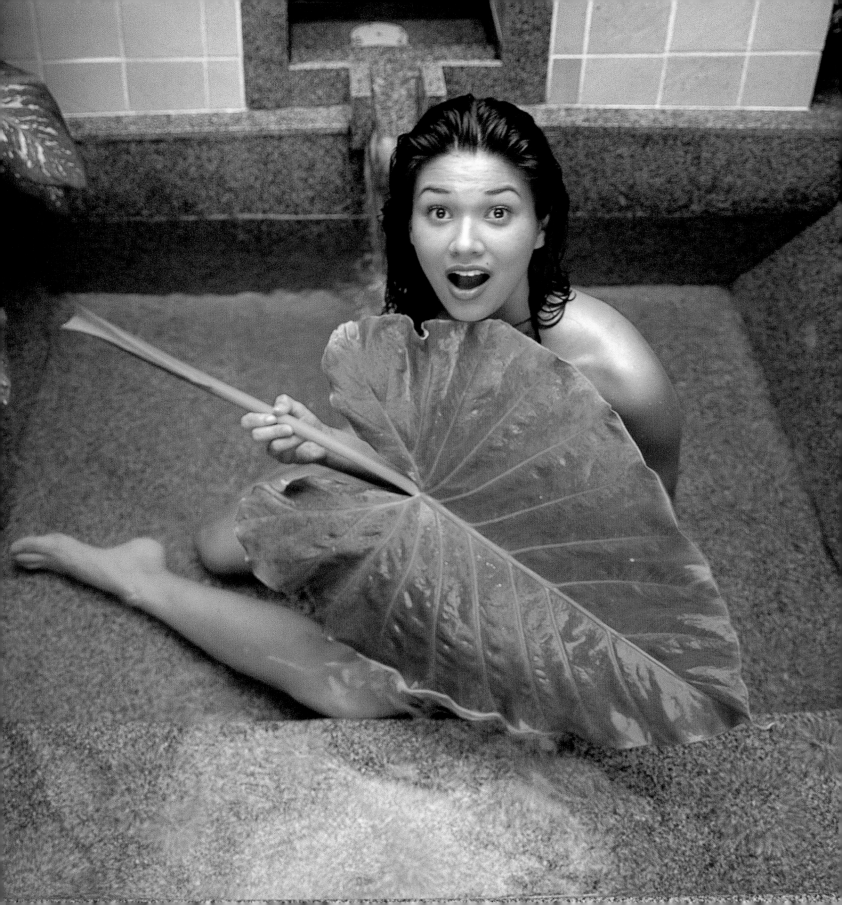

body conscious

Long limbs and vital statistics are minor contributors to the beautiful body. Much more important is the state of mind that sits on top. While there is barely a woman alive who is content with her natural shape, every woman can improve her body by upping the respect that she pays to it. This is achieved by taking time for herself – a vital part of life that most of us ignore.

The Asian approach to achieving and maintaining a healthy and beautiful body is a sensible one. For a start, it has no time for fad diets and punishing stomach crunches! Traditional body treatments from the tropics outstrip those from everywhere else in the world in number and variety and all of them rely on nature's own pharmacopoeia to produce results. Certainly not skin deep, they not only cleanse and soften our skin,

but also draw out impurities from within. Their ritual of application (especially at the hands of dedicated therapists in a spa context) relaxes us, empties our minds and soothes our souls in an atmosphere of peace.

All this emphasizes the oriental philosophy that regards beauty as a holistic concept embracing both the inner and outer self. For example, there are everyday words in the Indonesian language that are part of the more specific lexicon of body care which have no real equivalent in English. Indonesian women talk about having a *lulur* or *mangir* or *mandi susu* as readily as westerners talk of taking a shower. This chapter reveals some of the more exotic body treatments, be they scrubs, baths, wraps, heat treatments and polishes, for glowing skin... and improved self-esteem!

Mandi Susu

The tale of Queen Cleopatra and her milk baths is well known, yet do you know anyone who pours a few pints into the tub before climbing in? Trust the Indonesian people with their deep grasp of the good of the natural, to have their own form of milk bath. Known as *Mandi Susu*, it has soaked Javanese princesses for centuries as an elixir of eternal youth. Milk, from a goat, sheep or cow, makes skin radically soft and pure to the touch.

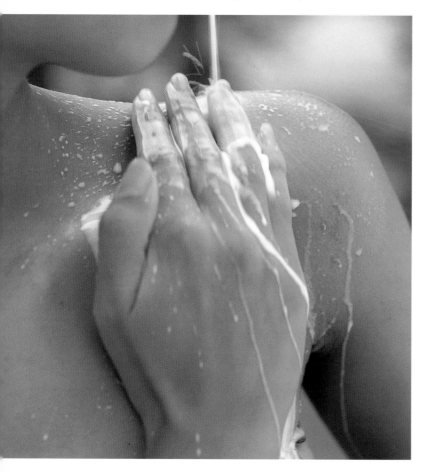

Modern formulations of this popular ritual have eliminated the taste and smell of milk while maintaining its nutrients with softening proteins. The *Mandi Susu* is a sought-after bathing ritual at the *St Gregory Javana Spa* in Singapore where therapists leave you soaking in a cloudy white tub for 20 minutes and advise you not to rinse afterwards. At home, you can pour fresh or powdered milk in with the bath water. Or for superior baby-soft skin, try natural yoghurt or buttermilk, but be ready to hold your nose!

Ocean Bath

This bath focuses on the healing properties of unrefined sea salt harvested on the east coast of Bali. Although not strictly thalassotherapy, this bath relies on the nutrients in the salt to draw out toxins from the body. The benefit of sea salt is based on the premise that sea-water has practically the same chemical make-up as human plasma allowing the body to easily absorb its healing properties.

The Ocean Bath at *The Spa at Jimbaran*, Four Seasons Resort, Bali is altogether a more exotic affair. Not only are the pure sea salts mixed with Bali Sunset Oil containing coconut, vanilla and citrus blends to uplift the senses, this hour-long treatment kicks off with a scalp, neck, shoulder and back massage. As if that were not enough, it takes place in the privacy of your own villa, where the bath tubs have earned an international reputation for their depth, size and comfort.

Floral Bath

For those of us born outside tropical Asia, the floral bath is the nub of the 'tropical spa' experience. We can hardly believe our eyes when a bucket of vivid blooms is tossed into the water purely for our pleasure. It is a sybaritic moment when the velvety petals tickle our bare skin. Flowers – jasmine, gardenia, tropical magnolia, hibiscus, frangipani, bougainvillea, poinciana, rose, globe amaranth, alamanda and ylang-ylang – are chosen both for their fragrance and rich colours.

In line with tropical mores, Asians believe flowers are the tangible link to the forces of the spiritual world, representing a symbolic purge of our earthly impurities. In Asian spas, the Floral Bath is not usually offered as a treatment on its own. It is often used as the finale to one of the many tropical body treatments on the menu. It becomes an opportunity to savour the cleansing experience and relax for a further 20 minutes or so.

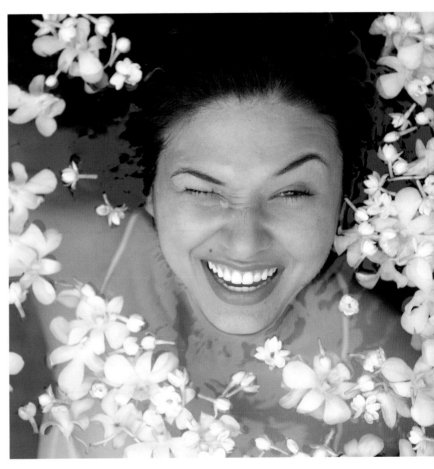

Aromatherapy Bath

The bath is a perfect place to enjoy the sensual pleasures of aromatherapy oils. Simply drop one or a combination of essential oils into warm water and spuddle. Some of the oils' properties are absorbed into the skin while the rest evaporate into the atmosphere for inhaling, simultaneously soothing muscles and mind.

A Few Recommended Bathtime Blends
Use up to ten drops of these essential oils either together or separately.

For calming	camomile, lavender, rose
For detoxifying	ginger, sage, rosemary
For passion	ylang-ylang, geranium, sandalwood
For brain boosting	grapefruit, lemon, mandarin, peppermint, pine

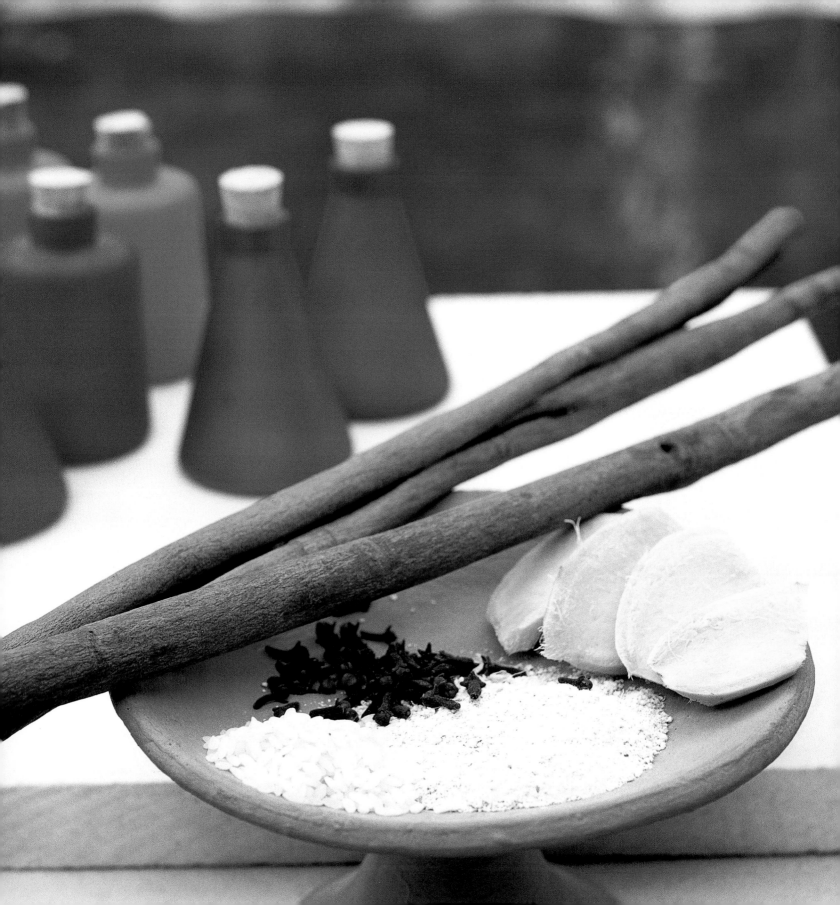

Balinese Boreh

If you reach for the Vicks pot at a hint of a chesty cough, this body scrub is for you. Out of all the oriental treatments the Balinese Boreh offers the most potent sensation – an all-over deep heat experience. The scrub is purely and simply a herb and spice mix: It is a centuries-old village recipe using spices we more readily associate with curry, and is prepared to warm the body at the first sign of windy weather.

As a tropical people, the Balinese live in fear of the cold and the health problems it can bring, so the whole family has a *boreh* both as a curative and preventative treatment. It feels really hot; it's good for fever, headaches, muscle aches, arthritis and chills. It increases the blood circulation and its exfoliating ingredients – cloves and rice – soften the skin.

The *boreh* is not recommended for pregnant women as the penetrative ingredients direct the heat away from the womb area to the body's extremities.

While most Balinese spas offer the *boreh*, this recipe comes from the *Nusa Dua Spa*.

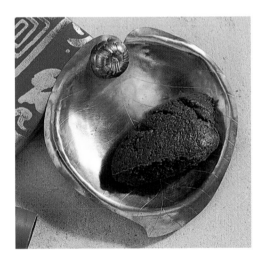

Ingredients
20 gms (4 tsp)	sandalwood
10 gms (2 tsp)	whole cloves
10 gms (2 tsp)	ginger
5 gms (1 tsp)	cinnamon
10 gms (1 tsp)	coriander seeds
10 gms (1–2 tsp)	rice powder (finely ground rice)
5 gms (1 tsp)	turmeric
10 gms (1 tsp)	nutmeg
10 gms (1 tsp)	lesser galangal water or spice-blended oil
3	large carrots, grated

The first eight ingredients are ground together in a pestle and mortar or bought prepared in powder form or dried in balls.

Steps
1. Add a little water or a spice-blended oil to the herb and spice mix to make a thick paste. For those who cannot tolerate a strong heat sensation, mix a greater proportion of ground rice powder to reduce intensity.
2. Cover your body; leave for five to ten minutes; feel the heat!
3. Rub the skin vigorously so that the mixture flakes away.
4. Gently rub the grated carrot into the skin. This replenishes moisture after exfoliating.
5. Shower and moisturize.

Traditional Lulur

The queen of treatments literally, this spice and yoghurt exfoliation and body polishing process has been practised in the palaces of Central Java since the 17th century. There, the pursuit of beauty has long been a daily ritual and the Javanese Lulur an integral step, leaving skin soft, supple and shining. Today, the Javanese Lulur (*lulur* is Javanese for 'coating the skin') is more usually administered each day during the week prior to one's wedding day. This stems from the belief that a bride should be at her most clean and pampered in preparation for child bearing – her first and foremost duty as a married woman.

This *lulur* is on the menu at all Indonesian spas offering 'traditional' treatments; it includes a massage, a spice-wrapped and yoghurt-coated body blitz, and a blossom-filled bath. It is an aromatic experience and lovely for all skins, although, if you're having difficulty choosing a body treatment, this one responds best to younger skins. The turmeric content can turn skins temporarily yellow, but generally this is a favourite, all round body treat.

For a traditional *lulur* that really makes you feel like a princess, the *Pita Maha Private Villa Spa* in Ubud, Bali, offers an hour and a half treatment using this recipe.

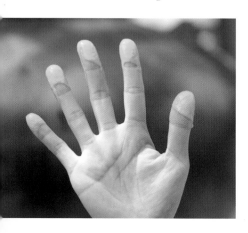

Ingredients

small bowl	a favourite body oil
30 gms (2 tbsp)	rice powder (finely ground rice)
10 gms (2 tsp)	turmeric
5 gms (1 tsp)	sandalwood
3 drops	jasmine oil
splash	water
500 gms (2 cups)	natural yoghurt
handful	a selection of fragrant flowers like rose, jasmine, ylang-ylang, frangipani…or whatever you like.

The rice powder, turmeric and sandalwood are ground together in a pestle and mortar or bought packaged as a powder.

Steps

1. Massage your body with your favourite oil.
2. Pulverize the spicy ingredients into a brown, granular paste, with a splash of water, and smear onto your body.
3. Once dry, gently rub the paste off the body in order to exfoliate and polish the skin.
4. Rinse your body under the shower.
5. Splatter your body with natural yoghurt using your hand to cover all crevices. Yoghurt contains a form of lactic acid that restores the natural pH to your skin and moisturizes it.
6. After rinsing, soak in a warm, flower-filled bath. Petals float over your body and the scent envelops you in a floral haze.

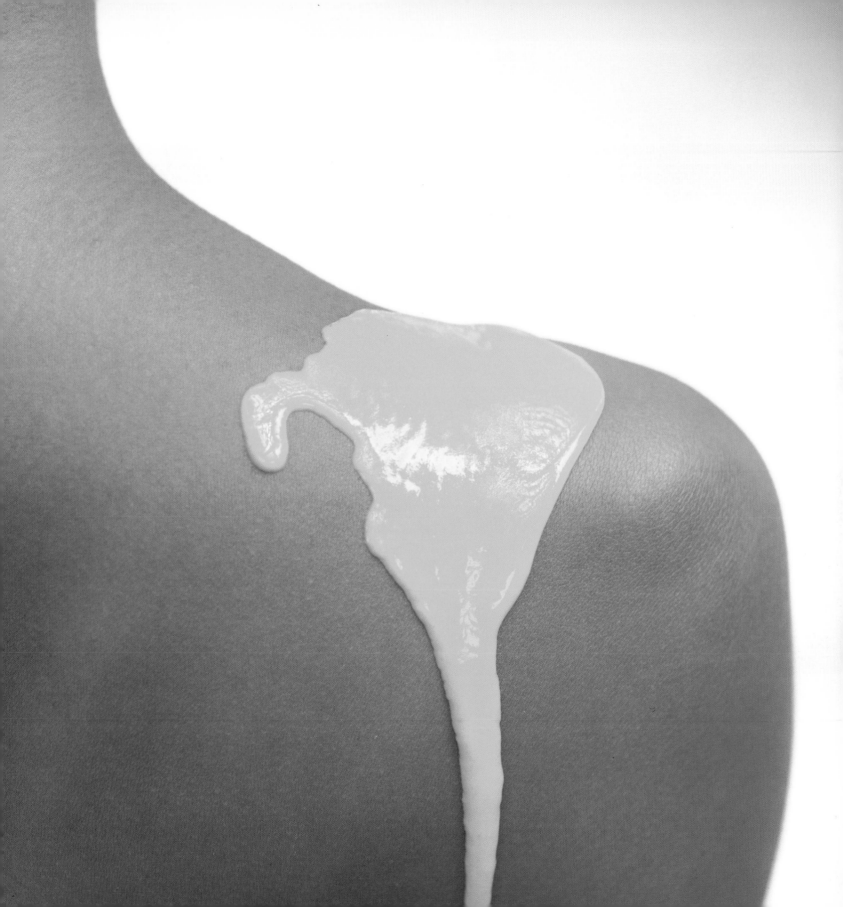

Volcanic Clay Body Scrub for Cellulite

Sadly there is no quick fix for beating that orange peel look that decorates the thighs of 95 percent of women. Improved diet, drinking water, dry skin brushing, swimming and yoga all help. And luckily the volcanic island of Bali is home to mineral-rich clays, which seep into the skin to break down those fat cells that are packed in a mattress effect underneath. A good cellulite treatment is the Volcanic Clay Body Scrub at the *Nusa Dua Spa*.

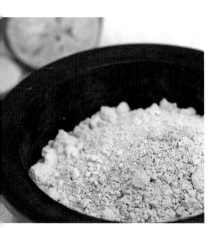

Ingredients

25 gms (2 tbsp)	Balinese clay (or any clay with purifying properties)
30 gms (2 tbsp)	sea salt
	water

Steps

1 Mix ingredients together, adding a little water to make a light paste.
2 Wipe cursorily over entire body. It leaves a thin, white film and feels prickly as it penetrates the skin.
3 Once the paste is dry, rub the skin so that it is sloughed away.
4 Shower and massage. The best essential oils for cellulite are nutmeg and rose. Add a few drops to a carrier oil or your favourite body cream, and apply liberally.

Cucumber Wrap for Sunburnt Skin

Feel the heat seep out of your sunburnt body using cucumber and essential oils. The best Cucumber Cooling Wrap is offered at the *Spa at Bali Hyatt*. Here's their recipe.

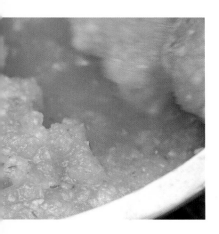

Ingredients

2 kilos (4 lb)	cucumbers, plus skin and pips, whizzed in a blender
2 drops	lavender oil
2 drops	tea tree oil
2 drops	camomile oil

Steps

1 Cover your body with the cucumber mixed with the essential oils.
2 Wrap the body in a gauze or cotton sheet; leave for 30 minutes.
   The cucumber feels cool on tender skin and you can sense the heat being drawn out of your body.
3 Cucumber leaves the skin soft, so moisturizing afterwards is optional.

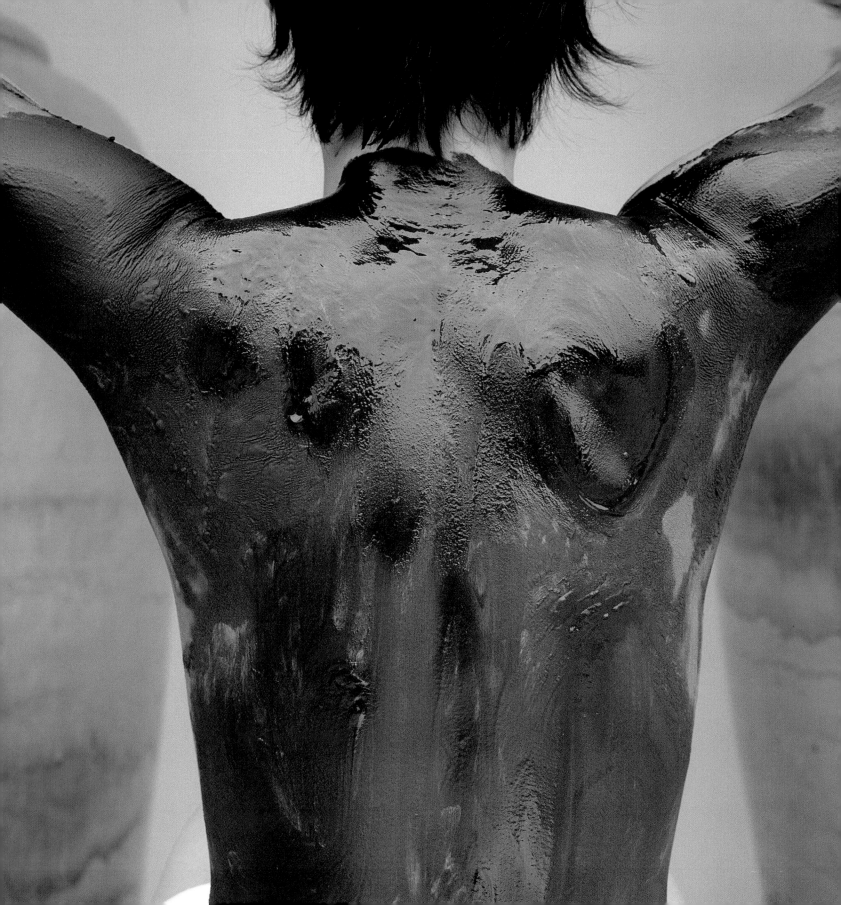

Thai Herbal Wrap

Enjoy this soft and aromatic body wrap only in Thailand where the healing properties of the country's mineral-rich mud remain both a mystery and a secret.

For a particularly seductive herbal wrap, which looks and smells more suitable for the dinner table than the body, visit *The Oriental Spa*, Bangkok. Here the hotel chef mixes a closely guarded recipe of white Thai mud, milk and turmeric, herbs and sesame oil which smells divine and feels soft and silky when applied to the skin.

Your body is wrapped in a plastic sheet, topped with towels while the creamy Thai mud concoction draws out any infection and impurities from the body and heals blemishes on the skin's surface. After perspiring gently for 20 minutes, take a shower, pat dry and feel the smooth, satin texture of your skin. There is no need to moisturize.

Alternatively the magic mud mixture used for the wrap at *Chiva-Som* (opposite) is dark and viscous like treacle. It feels warm and velvety on the skin and likewise is applied over the entire body, which is wrapped in a plastic sheet and covered with towels. This mud comes from the north of the country and is mixed with turmeric, marjoram and natural spring water.

Din So Porng (White Thai Mud)

Before the advent of deodorant sticks and Evian water sprays, the Thai people had a natural buster for body heat. They smeared mud all over their skins in order to tolerate their year-round hot and humid climate. The famous *din so porng* (white mud) is Thailand's traditional answer to an SPF. Its alkaline balance cools down the skin and replenishes moisture to prevent sun damage and subsequent skin disease.

However, like many of tropical Asia's natural remedies, *din so porng*, turns out to be an all-body panacea: it prevents perspiration, reduces fever, heals wounds, clears rashes and retains the skin's healthy, natural glow, as well as acting as an all-over cooler.

The mud, with its gypsum mineral content, can be applied in its natural state. But being the alchemists they are, Thai people commonly mix *din so porng* into scented balls with pollen and bark which they smoke in a fragrant talcum powder. These are simply crushed and applied for the ultimate skin food. Alternatively they can be combined with some specific perfumes for scented skin, or used as a body scrub to combat skin disease – even repair puss-infested wounds!

Mandi Kemiri for Mature Skin

If your skin tends to be a bit rough and leathery, you'll go nuts for a *Mandi Kemiri*, which literally leaves it glowing and feeling like silk. The pale, round *kemiri* or candlenut oozes so much oil that when crushed, it both exfoliates and deeply moisturizes the body. This luxuriant skin scrub is exclusively offered at *Jamu Body Treatments* in Jakarta and *Jamu Traditional Spa*, Kuta, Bali.

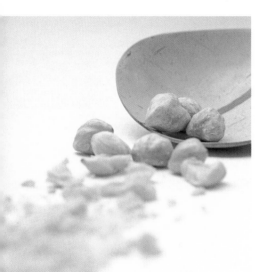

Ingredients

10 pieces	peeled candlenuts
a few shavings	galangal (can substitute with ginger or omit)

Steps

1 Grind the nuts coarsely in a pestle and mortar and add the white ginger so that the mixture looks and smells vaguely like crunchy peanut butter.
2 Rub gently over the entire body and then rub harder with the palm of your hand. The nut oil extracts dirt from the skin's pores so that when the scrub sloughs off with rubbing, the granules, which started out as a taupe colour, have turned dark with dirt.
3 Rinse under the shower. If you like the oily feeling on the skin, which is neither heavy nor clogging, don't use soap. Enjoy the lingering nutty aroma.

Coconut Body Glow for Sensitive Skin

Some 60–70 percent of women believe they have sensitive skin; if you fall into this category, try one of nature's treats: freshly shredded young coconut (rich in nutrients but not over-abrasive). The *Mandara Spa at The Chedi* in Bali offers this scrub using nutritious coconuts from Sulawesi.

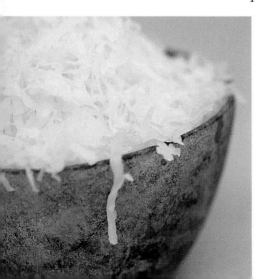

Ingredients

half	young coconut, freshly grated
1/4 tsp	turmeric powder (or 1 cm tumeric root, grated)
1/4 kilo (1/2 lb)	carrots, grated or blended
2 tbsp	gelatin, already set

Steps

1 Mix the freshly grated coconut with the turmeric (the latter is used for its cleansing properties and high vitamin C content).
2 Gently rub the mixture all over your body.
3 Leave for five minutes and wipe off with a wet, warm cloth.
4 Mix the carrot and gelatin and apply to the skin. This adds conditioning nutrients to the skin after the exfoliating process.

Papaya Body Polish

This erotic-sounding elixir has become synonymous with *The Oriental Spa* in Bangkok. Around the world people talk with titillation about their puréed papaya, smeared into all the body crevices which are left to sweat under a plastic sheet. Papaya contains certain enzymes, biochemically known as papain (it is used as a meat tenderizer) which soften and revitalize the skin when absorbed. The papain also settles the stomach, making it one of the best things to eat for an upset tummy. It is also perfect as baby food.

At home use ready-to-eat rather than unripe papaya (as the acid is too strong), purée it and spread it everywhere, without rubbing. Allow your body to sweat by rolling yourself up in a plastic sheet for 20 minutes. Wash off and feel the results!

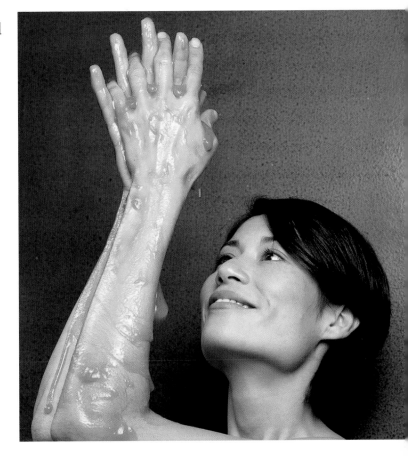

Just as Cleopatra used to bathe in sour milk to keep her skin smooth, tropical Asian women daub mashed, ripe papaya around their eyes to keep their wrinkles at bay. Due to the fruit's mild exfoliating properties, the skin loses a layer and wrinkles appear less noticeable. The enzyme contained in papaya works like an alpha hydroxy acid (a natural fruit acid that acts to remove the flaking cells on the skin's surface) without the tendency to cause skin irritation.

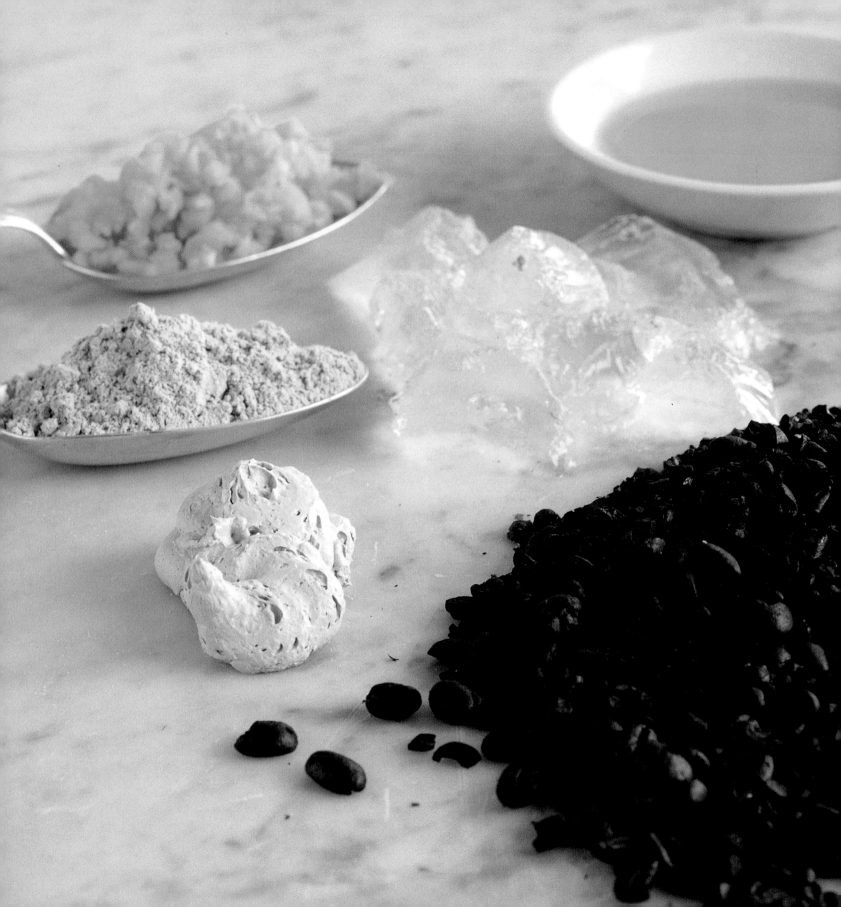

Bali Kopi Scrub

If you swoon when you pass a city coffee bar, imagine *that* smell for a full 45 minutes while the most fragrant of blends is smothered all over your body. Admittedly this coffee body scrub was only recently invented to cater for our addiction to the aroma of freshly ground beans. In Indonesia, where this scrub is offered, people stick to drinking the stuff, less as an excuse to sit and chat and more to give them energy while they work.

This scrub, rougher than some and ideal for male skin, is offered at all Mandara Spas (at *The Chedi, Ibah, Bali Padma* and *Nikko* in Bali), the *Novotel* in Lombok and Malaysia's *The Datai*) according to this recipe.

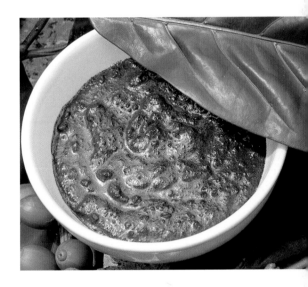

Ingredients

200 gms (6 oz)	Balinese coffee beans, ground
40 gms (3 tbsp)	kaolin clay (or cosmetic clay available at health shops)
pinch	ground pumice stone (optional)
1/4 kilo (1/2 lb)	carrots, grated or blended
10 gms (1 tsp)	gelatin, already set (optional)

Steps

1 Balinese coffee is the most fragrant of all Indonesian varieties, but you can substitute this for your favourite blend. Crush the dried beans quite finely and mix with the kaolin clay and ground pumice. Add a splash of water.

2 Rub over the entire body, later rubbing more vigorously so that the mixture sloughs off.

3 Rub the carrot, which can be mixed with the gelatin for easier application, into your body to replenish any lost moisture during the exfoliation process.

4 Shower and moisturize.

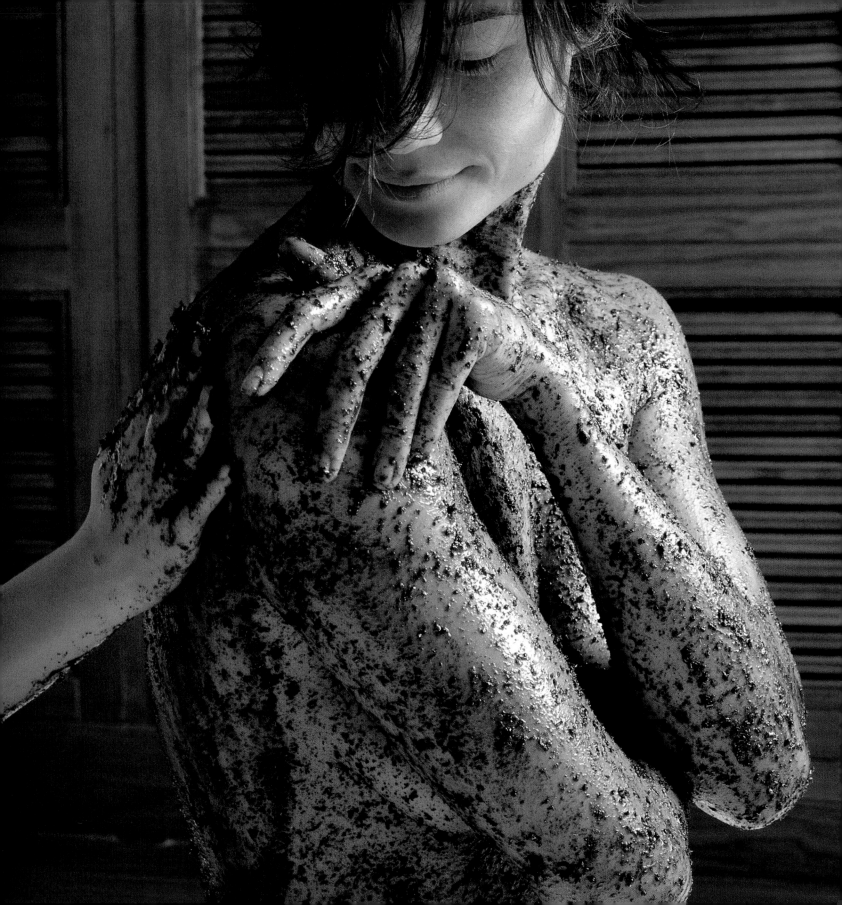

Oriental Body Glow

For the invigorating rather than relaxing route to soft skin, this traditional Thai body scrub is the way forward. It is on the menu at the *The Oriental Spa*, Bangkok and the *Banyan Tree Spa Phuket.*

Ingredients

1 cup	runny honey
1/2 cup	sesame seeds
sprinkling	dried herbs: lavender leaf, mint (which makes the mixture turn dark)

Steps
1 Mix the ingredients together and rub the thick, sticky paste over your body.
   Take your time so that the skin properly exfoliates and make the most of the sweet aroma reminiscent of that childhood smell of cooking caramel.
2 Shower. The whole process takes about half an hour.

Honey Treats

The humectant properties of honey nourish and moisturize the skin. You can use honey on both face and body. In Thailand, where it is produced under royal patronage in the north of the country, honey has traditionally been used to cover open wounds in order to soften scar tissue and encourage the growth of new skin.

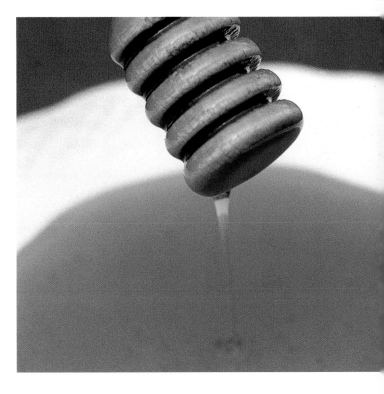

Face
1 Massage runny honey – with a squeeze of lime for astringent purposes or some ground oatmeal if you like a coarser texture – into damp skin for 15 minutes.
2 Rinse your face with warm water to leave it feeling soft and peeled.

Body
1 Cover body with honey and sit in the steam room.
2 Shower.
Such a gentle treatment can be used two or three times a week for normal to dry skin.

Thai Herbal Heat Revival

This heated muslin parcel of aromatic herbs and spices is a heavenly health treatment in the raw; it is unchanged since Thailand's Ayutthaya period (14th –18th century) when a fragrant hot-pack was administered to war-weary soldiers returning home with muscle aches and bruises.

Today the poultice is still used to alleviate pain or inflammation (especially good post partum) by opening the pores and bringing a medicinal heat to the muscles to induce relaxation.

The Thai herbal pack is excellent at *The Oriental Spa*, Bangkok and *Banyan Tree Spa Phuket*. For an authentic steamy session, to soothe sore muscles and relax, combine the herb pack with a massage at the Thai Massage School, located in the corner of the beautiful Wat Po temple in Bangkok. Watch out for some real heat here and some temporary yellow skin staining (from the turmeric), but leave feeling better than believed possible!

Fill the parcel with a random mixture of the following straight from the kitchen of *The Oriental Spa*, Bangkok:

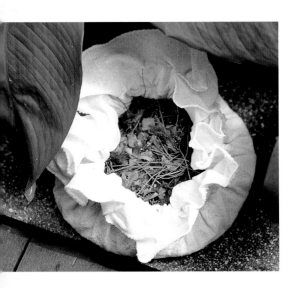

Ingredients

prai (common Thai herb)	for relief of sore muscles and tired joints
turmeric	an anti-bacterial skin freshener
lemon grass	an astringent for skin blemishes
Kaffir lime	for toning mature skin and for boosting circulation
camphor	for cleansing minor infections

Steps

1. Packed tight the parcel should be pomelo size, weighing roughly 400 gms (³/₄ lb).
2. The pack should be heated over a steamer or hot pot. It can be left steaming until needed, at least five minutes.
3. The poultice can be placed anywhere on the body for 30 seconds to one minute in each place. It should not be used on the face or genital area. It is good for slimming.

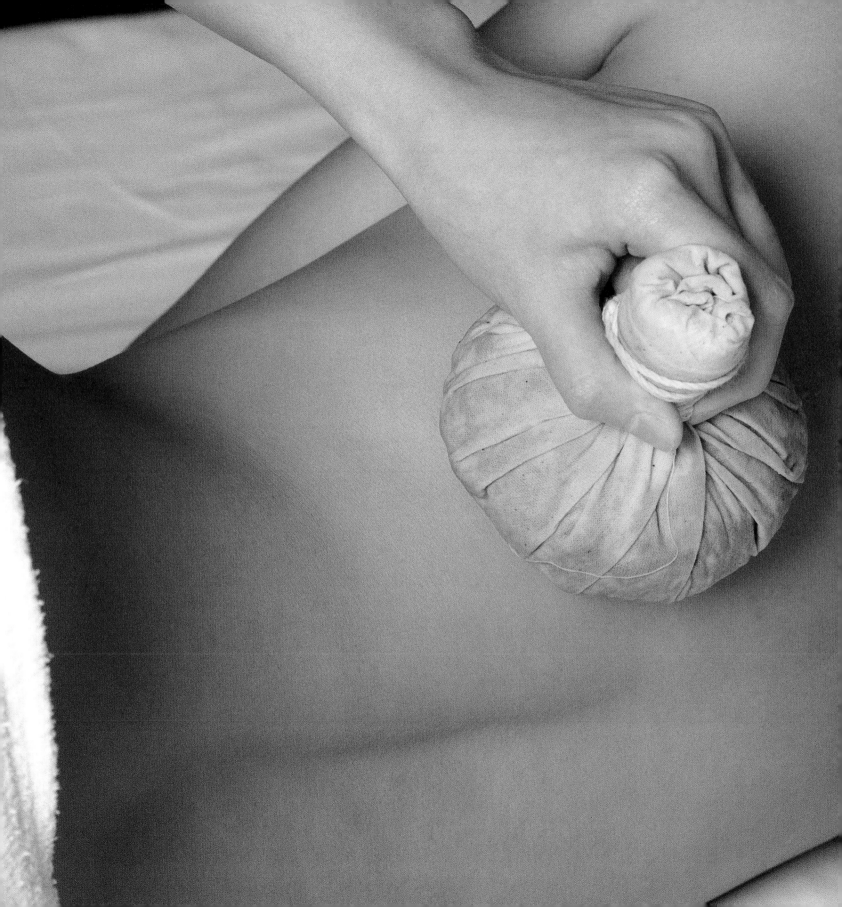

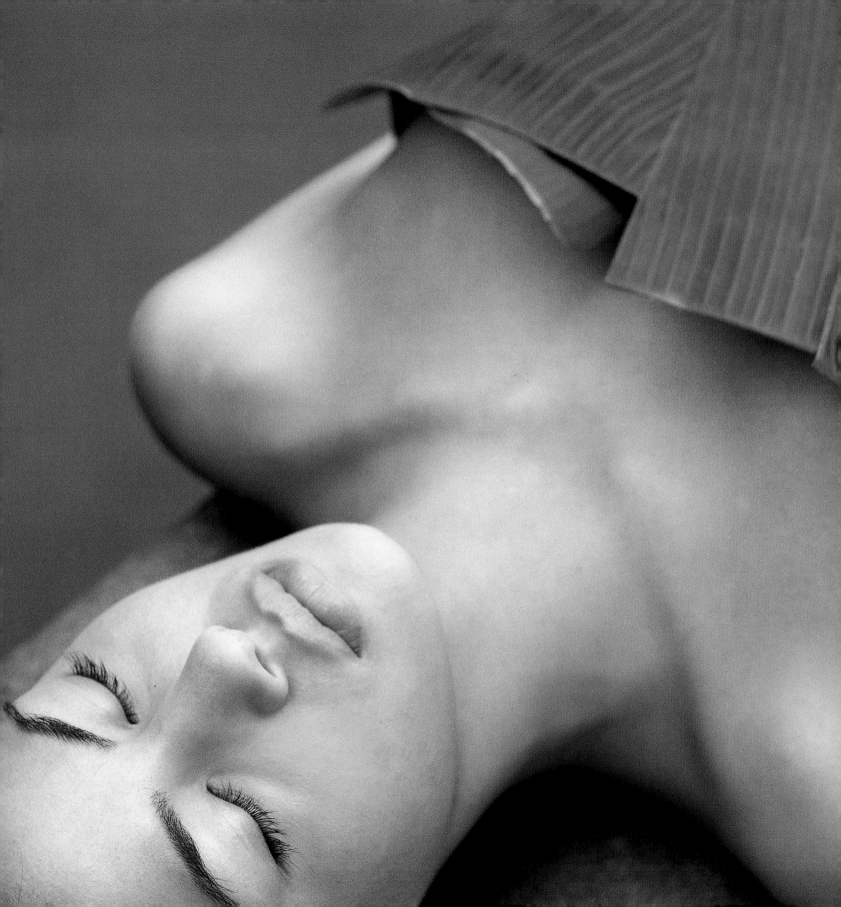

Aloe and Lavender Wrap

Aloe is grown and used in abundance in Indonesia, its long, spiny leaves cut and squeezed to release a sticky juice, ideal to pacify upset skin, stimulate the scalp and add fullness and lustre to hair.

While aloe is a major ingredient in all kinds of sensitive skin products, there is nothing more seductive than a coating of aloe, lavender and banana leaves, offered in this wrap at the *Spa at Jimbaran,* Four Seasons Resort Bali.

Ingredients

1 tsp	fresh aloe
to cover body	aloe vera gel (store bought)
a few spritzes	lavender essential oil mixed with distilled water
12 pieces	banana leaves (approximately 20 cm x 10 cm)
4	lemons or limes, cut in half
few drops	lavender essential oil
generous amount	lavender body lotion (or your favourite)

Steps

1   Stir the fresh aloe into the bought aloe gel and smear the mixture over the body, but first rub it between your palms to take off the chill. With a good gel, this feels wonderfully soft and slippery, rather than sticky on the skin.

2   Spritz the lavender essential oil in distilled water over your body for a heady fragrance.

3   Place the banana leaf patches over the top of your body and round your arms, so that all limbs are loosely covered. According to Balinese tradition you should not lie on top of banana leaves as this denotes part of the ritual that prepares a body for cremation. While banana leaves are not beneficial to the skin in themselves, they do help to take the heat from the body. They feel gentle and soothing on the skin without feeling cold. A cotton sarong can be placed on top to keep the leaves in position. Lie still for 20 minutes.

4   As the wrap is conditioning and relaxing the skin, this is the ideal moment for a head massage from a friend or loved one!

5   Remove leaves and shower; then douse your body with warm water infused with the juice of the lemons or limes and a few drops of lavender essential oil. Together these rinse and soothe the skin.

6   Finish with lavender body lotion.

Java Wrap

The Java Wrap is a global beauty phenomenon waiting to happen: an age-old process for a new-age answer to slimming. It started out as a 40-day ritual to rid the midriff from post birth bagginess and, even today, the Indonesian woman lovingly restores her body this way. It is believed that the Java Wrap helps flush out the bacteria which gather in the body after childbirth. It gets the lymphatic system going, reawakens the body's organs, and cleanses and heals.

New mothers can also benefit from the mineral and citrus paste that is smeared around the middle, then bound tight in a cotton corset. As the old saying goes: "you have to suffer for beauty". This figure-saving treatment is time-consuming rather than really uncomfortable, unless you visit the *St Gregory Javana Spa* in Singapore where all the work is done for you.

The special paste recipe is fairly standard throughout Indonesia where it has been handed down from one generation to another, and administered woman to woman in the household. This treatment is best done by one friend to another.

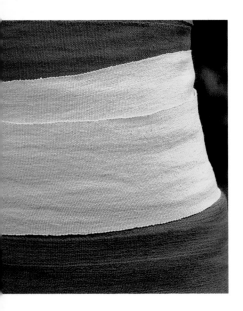

Ingredients

eucalyptus	strong antiseptic, benefits digestion
crushed sea stone/coral	calcium and other mineral content which warms and firms
fresh lime juice	an astringent which flushes toxins from the body
betel leaf	a leaf with antiseptic properties to cleanse womanly odour
massage oil	containing mint and eucalyptus essential oils for anti-viral and decongestant properties, also cooling.
cotton cummerbund	8–10 m long, 10–20 cm wide (8–10 yds long, 1 ft wide)

Steps

1 Mix enough ingredients to half-fill a cereal bowl with sufficient massage oil to give the paste a tacky texture that sticks to the body.
2 Rub the paste gently from above the tummy button to below the bottom.
3 Let it dry for 10 minutes, so that its healing properties start to soak into the skin.
4 Wrap the cummerbund neatly and tightly around the body starting under the bottom and weaving upward to the waist. The wrap physically constricts the body and helps to squeeze it back into shape!
5 Leave for 20 minutes, shower and moisturize with a gentle oil or lotion.
6 Post partum women in Indonesia also drink copious amounts of nourishing tonics such as turmeric, lime or betel leaf water.

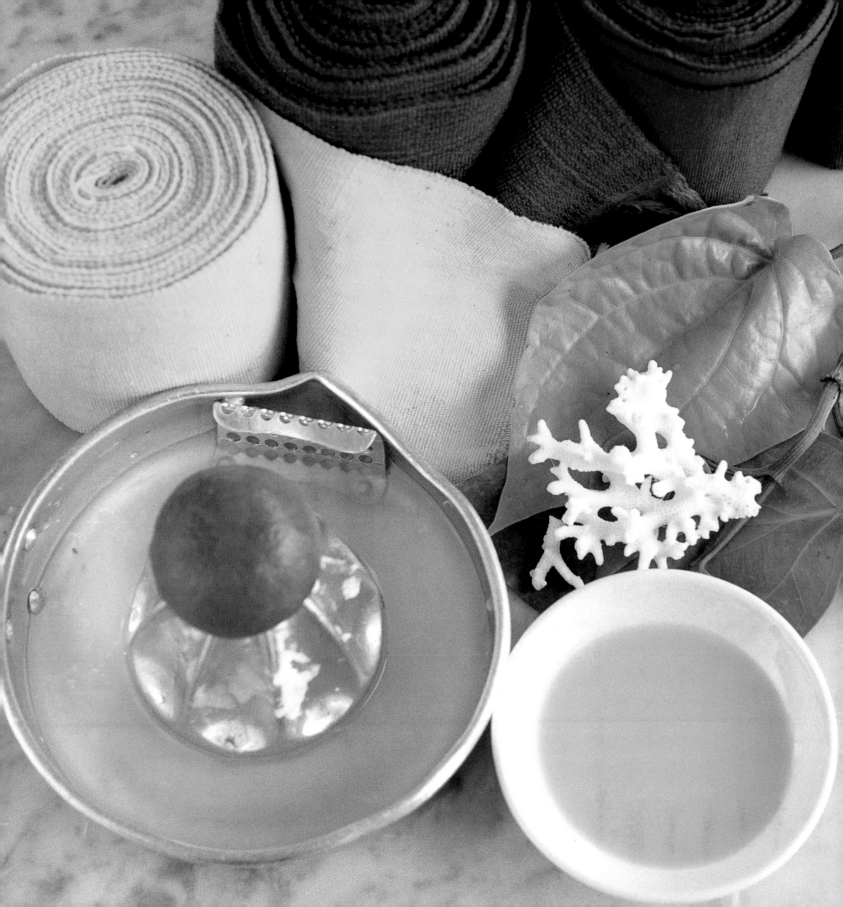

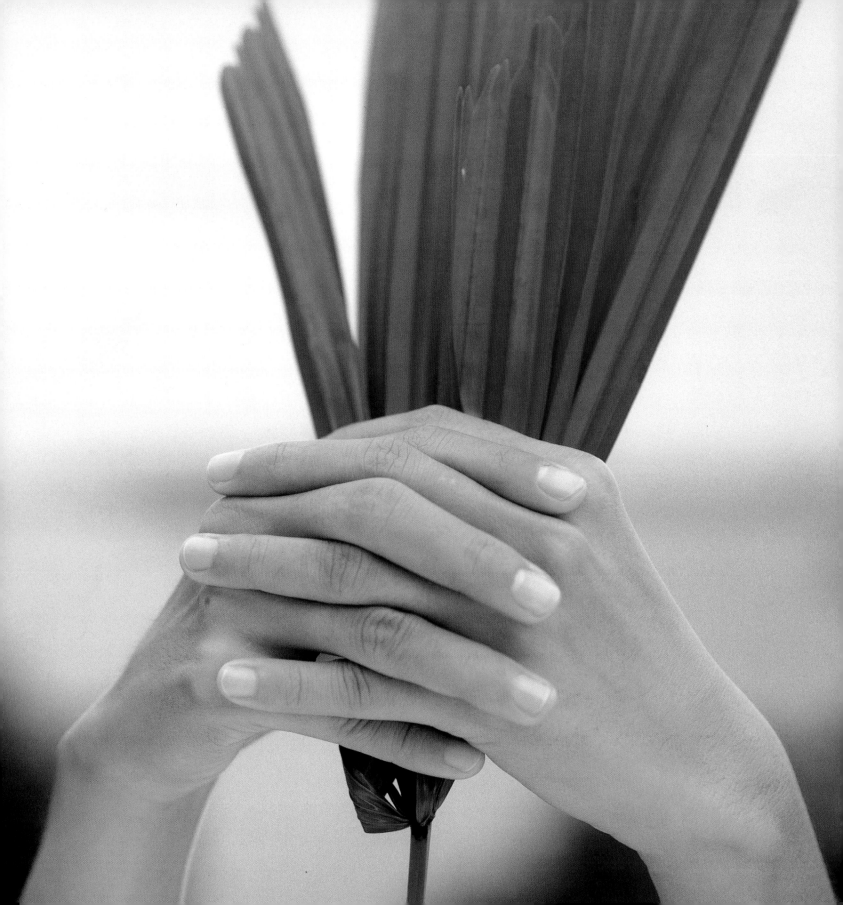

rites of massage

The power of touch is part of being human; it is part of our earliest awareness of being alive as babies in our mothers' arms. However, most people live in cultures that leave them isolated from one another. They give themselves no time to enjoy the simple pleasures of physical contact unless confined to the intimacy of the bedroom.

This is not the case in tropical Asia where massage is a part of everyday life from birth. Asian people understand that massage is all about sensual healing for the emotions as well as for the body, a simple and effective route to general wellbeing via our largest sensory organ – our skin. Skin is equipped with thousands of touch receptors; reacting to external stimuli, they transmit messages and sensations through our nervous system.

Massage is probably the oldest and simplest form of health care. It is depicted in Egyptian tomb paintings and mentioned in ancient Chinese, Japanese and Indian texts. It is thought to have originated in the East as a method for unblocking the *chi*, the vital energy flowing through our bodies that tends to get trapped due to emotional and physical upset. In Asia, massage has always been the backbone of health and wellbeing.

There is no mystery to the power of massage. The uncomplicated process of kneading, stroking and pressing the body is proven to unleash countless therapeutic benefits from the general: helping heart rate, blood pressure, breathing and digestion, to the more specific: aiding diabetic children, premature babies and cancer and HIV patients.

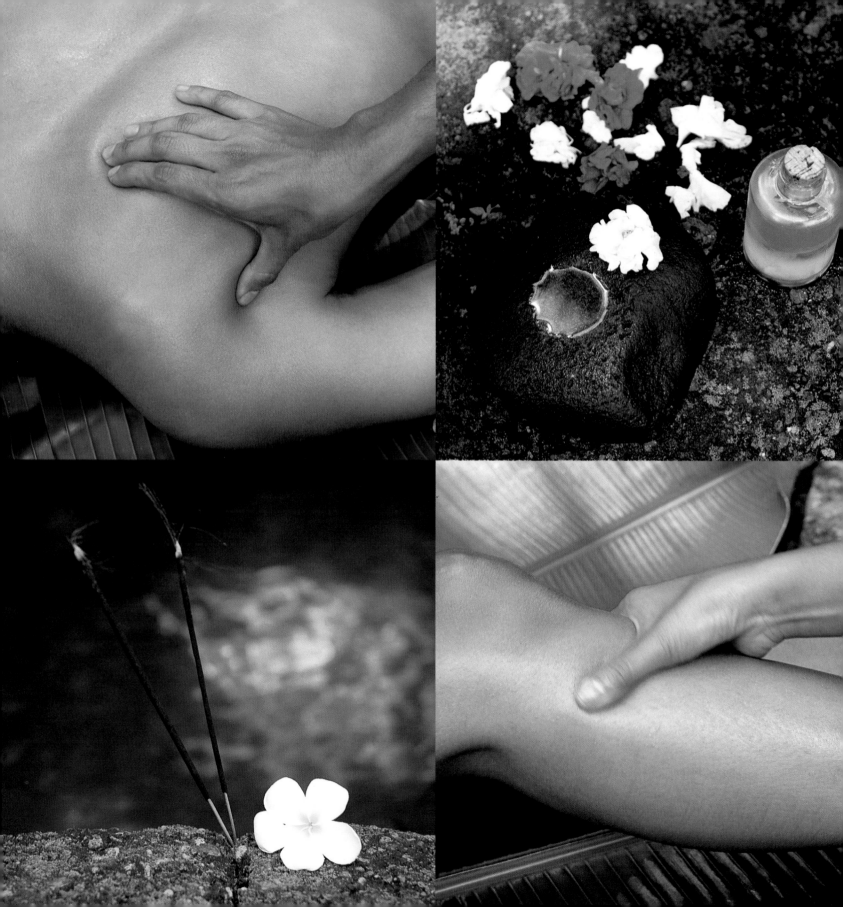

Traditional Indonesian Massage

We are creatures designed for touch. It is certainly the most personally experienced of all sensations. And the Indonesian people understand this better than most. Low-touch Western society keeps tactile expression behind closed doors, while Indonesians touch all the time: walking hand in hand and arm in arm, and stroking each other as a way of life.

They carry compassion in their hands. This they pass on naturally through massage to all the family from birth to death. Without a working knowledge of anatomy, many Indonesian people have an in-built sensibility to congested, tight or hot areas in the body, which they carefully relieve with the power of their hands and the application of aromatic oils.

It's interesting that Western culture, that has put so much faith in science for cures, and in medical practitioners for answers, is now turning, disillusioned, to touch therapies: Reiki, kineisiology, cranial osteopathy, aromatherapy, reflexology, all variations on a cure practised for centuries by Asian peoples.

Indonesian massage puts touch back into your system. As well as an unconditional desire to please and an intuitive reaction to the body, here is what to expect:

- medium pressure.
- scented massage oil: coconut oil prepared with local flowers such as champak (tropical magnolia), *akar wangi* (vetiver) and pandanus leaf is the traditional preparation; however, coconut is a heavy oil not suited to everyone, and is not always used in spas. (Balinese people chew on the white flesh, ingest the juices, spit out the fibres and rub them onto their skins for nourishment).
- long sensual strokes, working the length of the muscle to relieve tension. All sequences finish with upward strokes toward the heart.
- rolling skin between thumb and forefinger to spark up the nerve endings and increase blood flow.
- circular thumb movements for the same.
- pressure on the points in the foot and hand reflex zones.

Carrier Oils

Essential oils are too strong to be applied neat to the skin so when used in massage they should be mixed with a carrier or base oil, usually a cold pressed vegetable oil which has its own beneficial properties.

To obtain the correct proportions for a massage blend, add a number of drops of essential oil equivalent to half the number of millilitres of carrier oil. For example, for an average body size, pour 10 mls of carrier oil (or combination) into a bowl that is not plastic and add five drops of essential oil (or a combination of up to three oils).

Store massage blends in blue or amber glass away from sunlight to keep essential oils fresh. Vegetable oils should be used within 6–8 months before they turn rancid. Otherwise blend them with wheatgerm. Here are some of the oils most commonly used in an Asian tropical spa:

Almond

This vaguely aromatic oil is gentle and rich in proteins and vitamins. It is nourishing, light and softening for dry hands, eczema and irritated skin. It is a good lubricant, so blends well with other oils as an excellent massage base.

Avocado

This is a rich, heavy oil with high vitamin content. It is often blended for a velvet-like consistency. It also contains a mild sunscreen.

Coconut

Traditionally, this was the main carrier oil in tropical Asia because of its abundance. It is a thick saturated oil with its own distinct smell. It remains stable for a long period and is particularly nourishing in hair treatments.

Grapeseed

This is an extremely fine and pure oil, so light it absorbs immediately into the skin. It is good for helping the essential oils penetrate quickly. It leaves a satiny, not sticky, coating.

Jojoba

This is a natural fluid wax rather than an oil. It has a fine consistency (similar to collagen) which effectively penetrates the skin. It reputedly nourishes hair and prevents hair loss.

Macadamia

The acids in this oil are natural components of skin sebum. It has a rich nutty aroma and consistency. Its emollient qualities make it a good all round moisturizer, particularly for dry and mature skin.

Olive

Rich in proteins and vitamins, this oil is rapidly absorbed by the skin although it has a strong aroma and is often blended with other oils. It is a naturally warming oil, so it is good for massage in cold weather or in treatments for muscular pains.

Wheatgerm

This is a rich, dark oil, high in vitamin E but sometimes thought too heavy and aromatic to use alone. It is an antioxidant: it stabilizes essential oils and other carrier oils, making them last longer. It also benefits scarring.

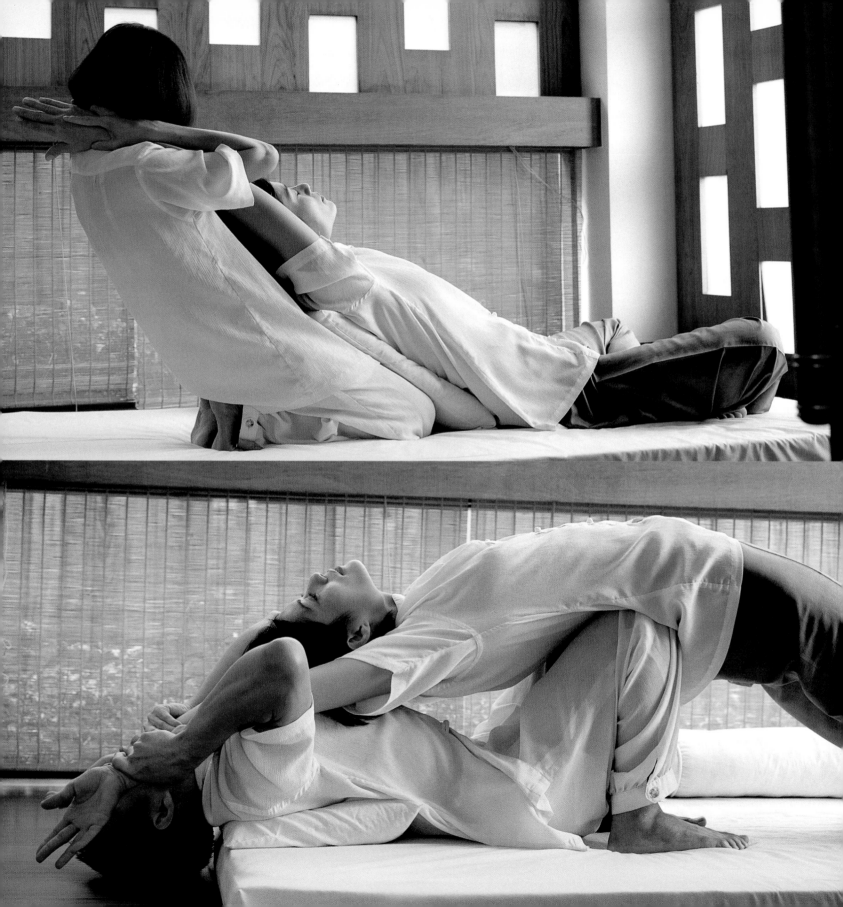

Thai Massage

It's the absence of oil and the addition of pyjamas that distinguishes Thai massage from all other massage therapies. Thai people claim that their skin is never dry enough, due to their country's hot climate, to need lubrication. They do, however, cover their bodies out of a sense of decorum in the face of some rather contorted positions! It is one of the ancient healing arts of traditional Thai medicine, the others being herbal medicine and spiritual meditation. Its style developed during the period of King Rama II out of the stretching techniques of Indian Ayurveda and the traditional Chinese focus on the body's pressure points. As a result, experts claim that Thai massage works more deeply than the more surface-oriented Swedish technique. It has an ability to heal, relax and realign the body.

By pressing on the body's energy meridians as well as its veins and muscle tips, Thai massage releases the sluggish flow of blood and build-up of toxins that gather in tired or overworked muscles. In a sense, it invigorates and heals them with a physical workout. This is combined with a spectacular technique, which mindfully stretches the limbs into positions that the uninitiated could never believe possible. Close body contact allows the masseur to hold, for example, the ankle in two hands, easing it away from the hips while pressing deep with his foot into muscles in the inner thigh. Such postures stretch the tendons and ligaments while making the body more supple, realigning it and releasing tension.

If this sounds more acrobatic than agreeable, be assured that good Thai masseurs, immersed in the 'middle way' of Buddhism, take a calm, meditative (not just physical) approach to their work, sensing the energy patterns in a person's body. Skilled therapists always start by softly squeezing the limbs with the palm of their hands in order to warm up the body and listen to its needs.

Important Body Parts in Thai Massage

Feet
Masseurs always start with the feet as this is where the whole body weight rests. Awakening the reflex points prepares the rest of the body for the massage.

Scalp
While nothing penetrates beneath the skull, massage along the scalp lines increases blood flow to the head where much of the body's tension is stored.

Ears
Masseurs spend a lot of time stretching and pulling these reflexology sensors, releasing headaches and helping with balance.

Face
A gentle fingertip pressure, Thai style, will release tension to increase blood flow and prevent wrinkles, while excessive pummeling will create them.

Essential Oils

The following essential oils are traditional to Southeast Asia. Best quality oils are extracted from plants (usually the leaves, flowers, roots or berries) through a process of steam distillation. As French aromatherapist Danielle Ryman points out: "extraction is a painstaking process as the amount of oil present in plants is minute."

Before the process of distillation, which has remained virtually unchanged for hundreds of years, people used medicinal plants in their lives by eating them, rubbing them onto wounds or making them into teas, poultices, tinctures and ointments.

Plants, flowers and their essences have played an integral role in healing disciplines in Asia and the rest of the world for thousands of years. 'Aromatherapy', as we know it today – the art and science of treating illness and emotions with essential oils – was formalized by a French chemist, Dr R M Gattefosse in the early 20th century.

The powerful properties of essential oils are best absorbed through the skin or through inhalation. Their aroma can eliminate blocks and restore body balance. They are great companions for the emotions they can ignite and help they can bring in promoting health and harmony in our modern lifestyles.

Clove

• This small evergreen tree originates from the coasts of the Moluccas in Indonesia but is now grown in most tropical climes. Its flowering buds turn into the familiar brown cloves when dried and these, along with the leaves, are distilled into the oil.
• A strong, woody base note with a sweet, spicy vanilla scent.
• Clove oil is an antiseptic and anaesthetic: a drop on a sore tooth will numb the ache. It is a general tonic for physical and intellectual weakness and is known to help overcome frigidity, claiming similar properties to opium. It is valued for its digestive properties, so when massaged into the abdomen, it relieves pain and diarrhea. Suck a clove if you are feeling stressed or wish to give up smoking. Infused into the atmosphere, clove will brighten the spirits.

Ginger

• The oil is distilled from the tuberous, pungent root of the tropical plant which originated in India but is now grown in many countries.
• A warm and spicy fragrance with a stimulating, almost lemon top note.
• Ginger is well known for its aphrodisiac qualities best administered by mixing with a base oil for massage in the lower spine. It eases muscular aches and pains and is therefore good for menstrual cramps. It relieves flu symptoms and its warming qualities help sweat out fevers and colds and treat digestive disorders.

Jasmine

• The fragrant white jasmine blossoms come from an evergreen shrub grown all over Asia. Jasmine symbolizes the sweetness of a woman and is the flower most used in perfumery: it reputedly takes more than 10,000 crushed heads to produce one ounce of *Joy*, Jean Patou's famous fragrance and one of the most expensive in the world.

• The aroma is sweet and euphoric.

• Jasmine uplifts the soul; it is used as a sign of friendship and as a Buddhist offering in Thailand. Indonesian women weave the flowers into newly washed and oiled hair to infuse it with perfume. It relieves pre-menstrual mood swings and pains as well as labour pains when applied as a compress. It softens dry skin and reduces stretch marks. It unearths compassion and inspires artistic creativity. Use the oil in a burner, in massage, or in the bath to feel seductive.

Nutmeg

• A sturdy evergreen tree that originated in the Spice Islands. The kernels of the fruits are the nutmeg, while its red lacy covering is mace. In cookery, it is used in cakes and curries.

• Warm and spicy with musky overtones.

• Nutmeg aids the digestive system by breaking down starches and fats. Used sparingly in massage oils, its warmth helps muscular aches and pains and stimulates the circulation. It is especially good to strengthen contractions in childbirth, and also has purifying properties.

Patchouli

• While patchouli is native to Malaysia, 450 of the 550-tonne annual world production comes out of Sumatra, Indonesia, from a small, fragrant shrub bearing white flowers, tinged purple.

• Strong, woody, wet and earthy fragrance.

• In the West, patchouli oil was favoured by the flower children of the 1960s for its flair for arousing sexual passion and psychic awareness. In the East, this oil is redolent of Bali where it is burned everywhere to create a relaxing atmosphere. Patchouli is great for skin conditions, mixed with oil for acne, eczema, burns and scar tissue.

Sandalwood

• The best sandalwood comes from plantations in Mysore, India. The oil is extracted from the roots and the centre of the slender trunk when the sandalwood tree is 50 years old.

• Syrupy, sweet, thick and heady aroma.

• Of all aromatics, sandalwood plays the supreme role in eastern religious ceremony, symbolizing spirituality. It is a major cosmetic ingredient, particularly in oriental perfume. Use it in massage oil to treat dry skin, in baths to relieve cystitis and infections, and in burners to calm the nervous system and promote clarity of thought. This is a particularly grounding and balancing oil.

Vetiver

• Vetiver oil comes from the roots of vetiver grass grown largely in India and Indonesia.

• Deep smoky base note, with a woody yet sweetly spicy undertone.

• Known as the 'oil of tranquillity' in India for its deeply relaxing effect, vetiver is traditionally woven into mats or screens and hung in rooms to evoke a sedative atmosphere. It keeps insects away, and while it stimulates blood flow and relieves muscle tension, it also stimulates the production of breast milk if massaged with oil into the chest. Like sandalwood, it is beneficial for anxiety as well as insomnia and helps you cope in times of upheaval.

Ylang-Ylang

• The ylang-ylang tree is known as the 'crown of the east' and the 'perfume tree' due to the overwhelmingly sweet smell of its flowers. It originated in the Philippines and is grown all over tropical Asia.

• Sumptuous and sugary fragrance with high notes like hyacinth and narcissus.

• In Indonesia the beds of newlyweds are scattered with ylang-ylang to proffer luck, harmony and fertility. Indeed, the oil is a famed aphrodisiac, most effective when dropped into bath water. By stirring the emotions, ylang-ylang resolves conflicts between partners and brings harmony, peace and warmth. It is good for nervous, stressed people and is an effective skin treatment and sun tanning aid when mixed with nut oils.

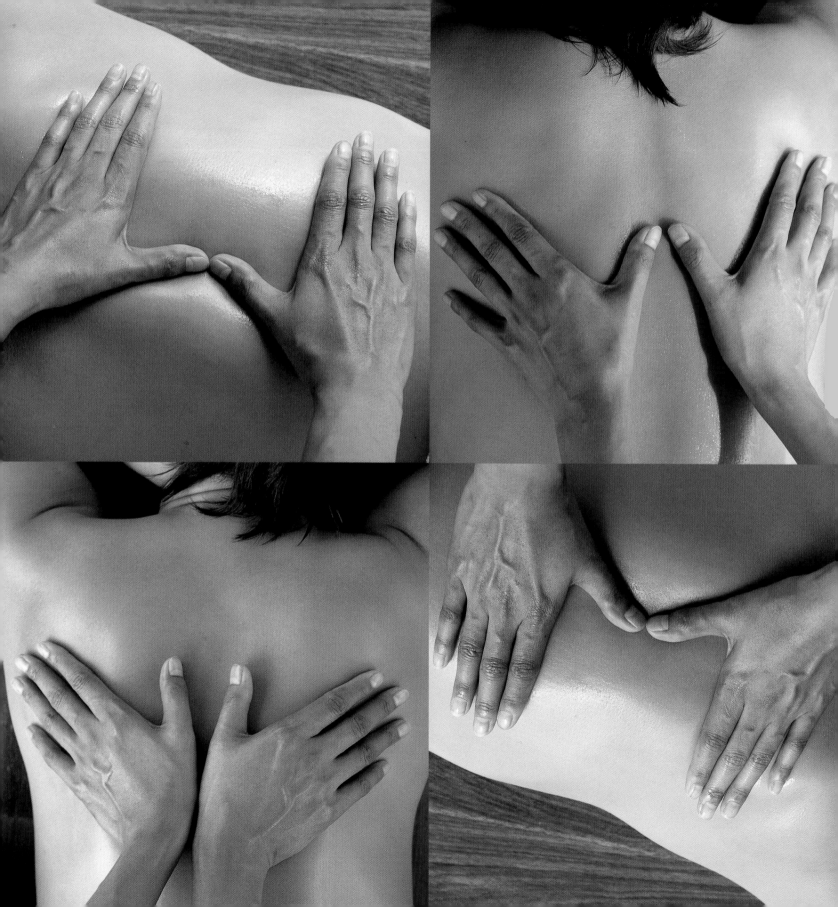

Aromatherapy Massage

Aromatherapy massage is one of the most popular treatments at a tropical spa. Although available throughout the world, its sensual experience is elevated to new levels in Asia thanks to the gentle and sensitive nature of its practitioners. Therapists appear to approach each and every massage as a bespoke, individual craft, rather than another body on their daily production line.

Through massage the active molecules of essential oils, already blended with a carrier oil, penetrate the bloodstream and soothe the central nervous system. For most people, the barrage of citrus, floral or spicy notes of the oils, like any smell, will bring back a stream of memories. The physiology of smell and emotion are supposedly closely linked. Apparently the olfactory sensors in our nasal passage can recognize up to 10,000 different aromas. In addition, as the massage activates the body's nerve endings and stimulates its blood flow, the medicinal properties of essential oils act on the internal organs and treat ailments. Although the oils only remain in the body for three or four hours before they are excreted, they have already triggered a healing process.

Mandara Massage

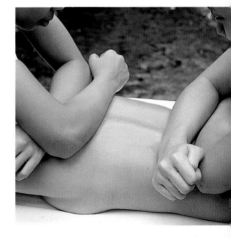

The Mandara Massage is the zenith of massage experience. This is thanks to the uncanny sychronization of two therapists who work together all over the body. The melodic rhythm of their strokes creates a pattern of sensation so pleasurable that you feel almost guilty for the indulgence. With one at the top and one at the toe, the therapists' hands move in harmony with each other, without ever leaving your skin. Their unique combination of six massage styles: Hawaiian Lomi-Lomi, Swedish, Balinese, Japanese Shiatsu, Thai and Aromatherapy ensures that every nerve ending is caressed. This is hypnotic, exotic and euphoric.

The Mandara Massage was exclusively devised for Mandara Spas (at *The Chedi, Ibah, Bali Padma* and *Nikko* in Bali, *Novotel* in Lombok and Malaysia's *The Datai*). It takes its name from the Mandara of Balinese legend – a mythical mountain that flows with eternal youth. Translated into an earthly equivalent, this massage is as close as one gets to such a sublime concept.

Tropical Oil Blends

Blending essential oils is an enriching part of aromatherapy. It opens up a Pandora's Box of fragrant opportunities. By composing your own blend you can strike the perfect note for your mood and discover your own way to sensual healing.

Many tropical spas and natural product companies have come up with their own scented oil blends to enhance the seductive nature of the various treatments for body, mind and soul. Here are some of the most inviting:

Peace of Bali Oil

Exclusive to the *Spa at Jimbaran*, Four Seasons Resort, this oil is a sacred blend of sandalwood, ylang-ylang and a touch of citrus. The combination has a calming and grounding effect just like the natural peace that Bali bestows.

Bali Sunset Oil

A splash of nutmeg essential oil adds warmth to any massage blend. This oil from the *Spa at Jimbaran*, Four Seasons Resort, focuses on nutmeg, with a touch of vetiver and lemon grass. It is used as a symbol of the warmth of the sun and the radiant sunset which is magnificent at this spot on the island's coast.

Bali Santi

Prepared according to traditional methods in Ubud, Bali, this oil from *Utama Spice* is a rich blend of coconut oil infused with vetiver, patchouli and other herbs for pure relaxation.

Java Oil

By *Esens*, this is a stimulating blend of eucalyptus and peppermint, traditionally used as an analgesic as well as a headache remedy. It is a good blend to use when slimming.

Bali Oil

From *Esens* comes a wonderful all-round blend named simply, redolent of the romance of the island where it was born. A coconut oil base is infused with pandanus leaf, champak flowers and vetiver according to an old village recipe for body and hair.

The *Scents and Elixirs* range of oil blends from *Essential* is used at *Nusa Dua Spa*:

Exotic Fruits

A blend of citrus essential oils for uplifting the spirit. It is redolent of the fruits and flowers that are seen everywhere in Bali on the myriad offerings to the Gods.

Sensual Flowers

This blend, dominated by the floral ylang-ylang oil, is reminiscent of Bali's many ceremonies and the abundant flowers they include. The significance of nature is so powerful for the Balinese that they believe the sweeter the flower the quicker their prayer will rise to heaven.

Desert Spice

A curative blend, heavy with ginger essential oil, warms the body and embraces the mood of the Spice Islands. Varieties of this oil have been used for centuries during the rainy season.

Oils enjoyed at *Mandara Spas* include:

Mandara Oil

The signature blend from *Mandara Spas* is an oil for romance. Its main ingredients are sandalwood and patchouli and it is also recommended for dry and scaly skin conditions.

Harmony Oil

Which speaks for itself. The blend of citrus fruits, canaga and other floral essences balance the body, mind and spirit.

Tranquillity Oil

A relaxing blend of vetiver, ylang-ylang and other calming essential oils that relax and warm the body.

Bali Santai Oil

A rejuvenating and gentle oil concentrated with mandarin essential oil, especially soothing for a pregnant mother.

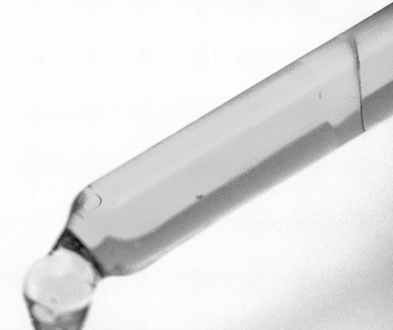

Rich and highly fragrant jojoba oil blends used at the *Spa at Bali Hyatt* include:

Stargaze Body Oil

Mixes cedarwood for stress reduction and a whiff of rose and orange to refresh and uplift.

Spirit Body Oil

Re-energizing oil that blends grapefruit for cell regeneration, lemon grass for muscle purification and lavender to calm the nerves so that you rise feeling recharged.

Sunset Body Oil

Best applied as an after-sun, thanks to the anti-inflammatory German camomile which soothes irritation. Together with sandalwood and lavender it has a sedating effect.

Moonlight Body Oil

Helps to gain balance in the body and stimulate cell growth if the skin has been sunburnt. This oil is a blend of frankincense which comforts, vetivert which has anti-inflammatory properties, sandalwood which strengthens the spirit and rose which is a balancing oil.

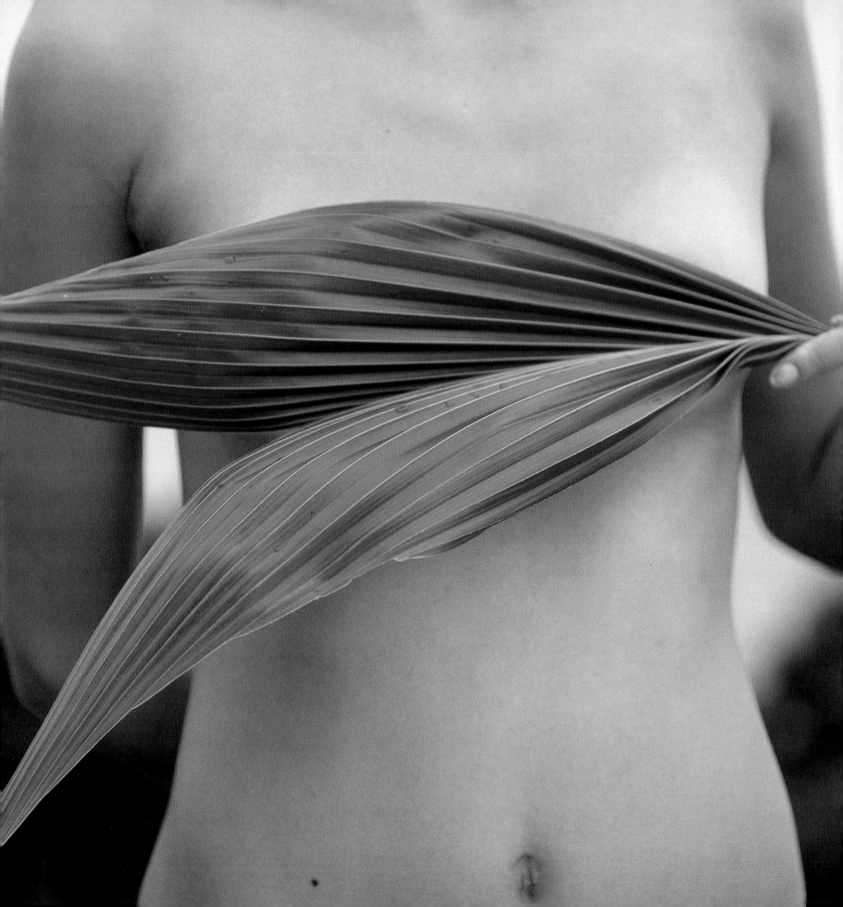

m i n d - b o d y - s p i r i t

There was a time, not so long ago, when the notion of beauty was literally skin deep. A costly cosmetic, where packaging was an artwork in itself, was the final answer to a smooth and clear complexion. It all ended here in the gold-topped tub.

Not any more. The materialistic '80s have given way to the caring '90s and a whole new approach to beauty that stems from within. It's the realization that it is not just our bodies but our minds and souls that need attention, if we are to be the radiant creatures that we all aspire to. Beauty no longer simply means a 'boob job' or a 'nose job', it means the pursuit of 'mindfulness', the latest buzz word for an overall sense of wellbeing that is deemed so important now.

In order to tap into this spiritual dimension, we are turning to mindful exercise – yoga, *tai chi*, meditation, even simple focused breathing techniques which offer physical and psychological benefits in one. All of this is a natural extension of the health and beauty treatments and the assault on all our senses which have come to represent the tropical spa philosophy. What is more: the mood for holistic self-preservation which has so recently become the favoured route to self-fulfilment in the West, has always been the unquestioned way of life in the East. Mindful exercise, in its varying guises, originated here in the simple belief that we can only look and feel good if our bodies and our spirits are working together in healthy harmony.

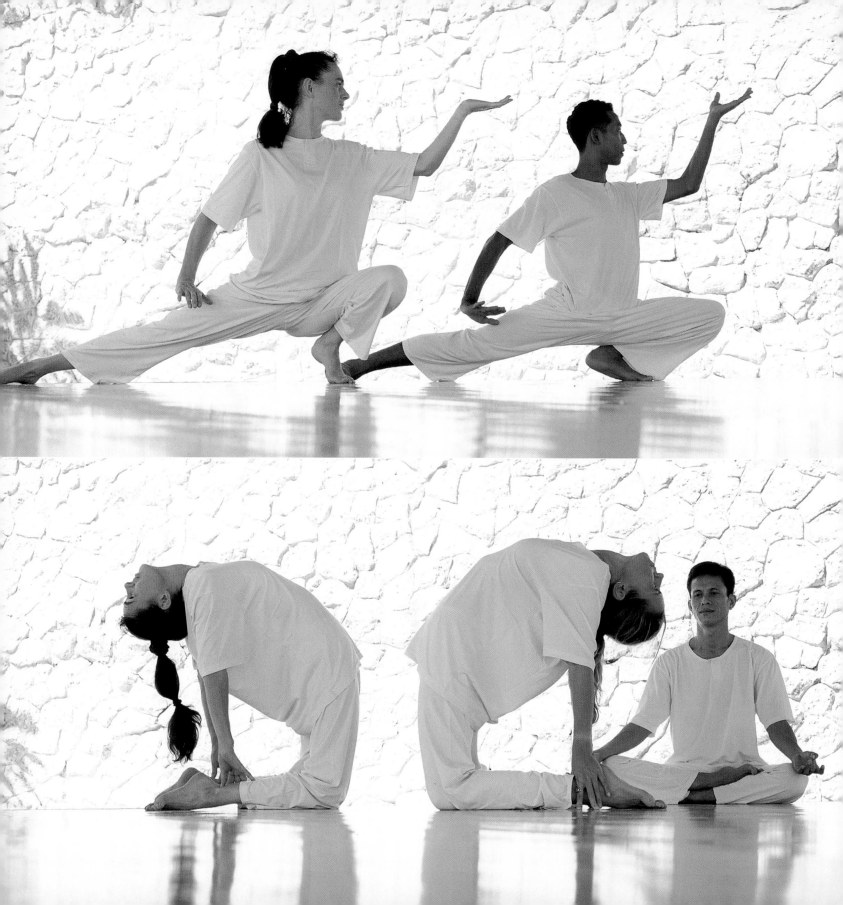

Tai Chi

This ancient Chinese movement therapy is all about harnessing the natural energy both within us and from outside. It relies on the belief that the smooth flow of *chi'* or life energy, through the body's meridians, is vital for good health and that illness occurs when there is an imbalance or sluggish flow in certain areas due to anxiety, tension and fatigue.

Tai chi is similar to yoga with its focus on breathing and its slow, meditative movements that concentrate our minds and encourage us to listen to that which we can never really hear: our inner self. However, *tai chi* has its own system of graceful arm movements that symbolize the deliberate process of harnessing the earth's energy and drawing it into our bodies. These movements, combined with strong leg postures, are learnt as a sequence practised time and again, although the sequence varies according to proficiency levels. Experts will practise the long version combining up to 108 movements in a 30-minute session.

Yoga

In its purest form yoga is a complete system of physical and mental training: a series of spiritual stages on the path to enlightenment dating back to 1200 BC in India when its wisdom and practice were passed down from Hindu ascetic guru to disciple.

The global spread of interest in yoga in the 20th century is unprecedented although much of its appeal lies in the catch-all benefits it unleashes: its ability to work on muscle groups, increase suppleness and vitality, tone internal organs, stimulate nerve centres, relieve stress and clear the mind. All this is attained through breathing techniques (*pranayama*) and physical postures (*asanas*) performed deliberately and slowly with a concentrated focus on our own inner awareness.

Yoga looks upon the body as the temple of the soul and in this respect is becoming a far more attractive alternative to the all-brawn-no-brain step class. Indeed exercise at its most seductive is a twilight yoga class under a Thai-style pavilion beside the beach at Thailand's *Chiva-Som* where the sea breezes and mantras help transport you to inner realms you never knew you possessed.

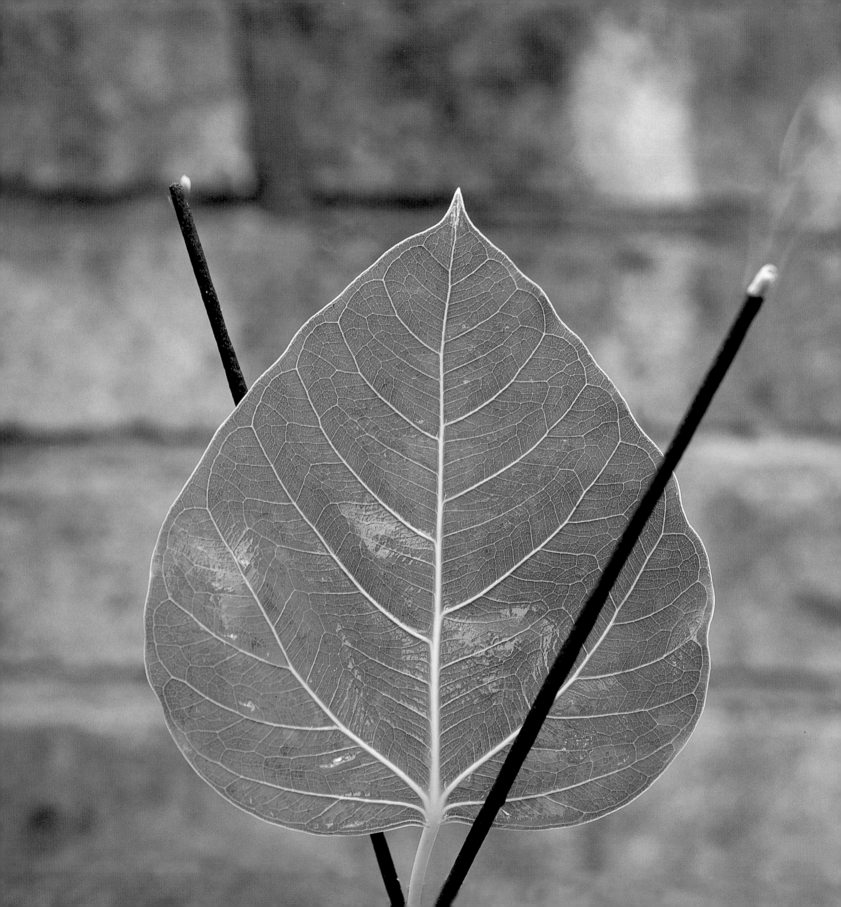

Meditation

It's all too easy to believe that meditation is a simple form of stress busting, that requires no physical workout and a bit of peace and quiet in which to breathe deeply and concentrate on 'nothing' in order to feel profoundly relaxed. For the uninitiated, this mental discipline is not so straightforward. It can be virtually impossible to drown out the incessant rabble of our internal dialogue and it takes practice to reach the state of heightened awareness and inner peace that meditation helps us to achieve.

The various techniques all involve focusing the mind on an object, colour or activity to which it can return if it gets distracted. These may include the conscious rhythm of breathing, a mantra – word or phrase such as 'Om', the most used and sacred mantra of the Hindus, or an icon such as a burning candle or religious statue.

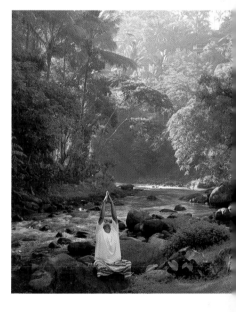

Once in a quiet, receptive state, the mind excretes certain brain waves, known as alpha waves, that purportedly operate at a far higher intensity than those that occur during sleep, creating electrical activity that leads to altered awareness and deep relaxation.

While different forms of meditation are practised in all major religions (in Christianity it takes the form of prayer), it is most readily associated with the spiritualism of the oriental world where it is used as a way of exploring the inner recesses of the mind and achieving a euphoric condition. This was picked up in the West during the 1960s when the Beatles popularized Transcendental Meditation (TM). By the 1990s, meditation in the West is no longer the preserve of the kaftan-clad fringe set, but has become an executive tool for beating stress, insomnia, addictions and depression.

It is best to be guided through the rudiments of meditation by a practitioner. However, some of the tranquil, tropical locations in Asia are so heavy with a spiritual silence that they provide a perfect sanctuary for getting started on the path to mindful relaxation. A location that immediately comes to mind is Sayan, outside Ubud in Bali, where sessions are offered at the *The Four Seasons* and *Begawan Giri Estate* by expert practitioners.

Yogaia Wave Movement

With so many forms of 'mindful' exercise currently in vogue, how do you choose what to focus on? Meditation clears the mind but doesn't do much for the cardiovascular and yoga is ideal as long as energy levels are not hitting the roof. This is where Yogaia Wave has found its niche. Called 'waving' by those in the know, this new exercise is a synthesis of forms that incorporates yoga, dance, martial arts positions and meditative practices, which together, bring a host of healing benefits. Who would have known that gyrating could do you so much good?

The co-founder of Yogaia Wave, Se'a Criss, is based at *Begawan Giri Estate*, Bali. She claims that this fun form of exercise realigns the body's physical structure, enhances the immune system, opens up the spinal column, balances the emotions and relieves anxiety – and, if this weren't enough – balances the left and right brain functions. Nevertheless, this is perfect for the 'mindful' exercise sceptic: it is a combination of aerobics without the schlep and yoga with a bit of pizzazz. In other words a complete mind and body workout.

Water Shiatsu Therapy

At last a grown up body treatment that makes us feel young again – really young. Water Shiatsu originated in America but has been developed as an aquatic body therapy for tropical waters by the *Breathing Space* in Singapore. It is so absorbing and comforting that it must – if only we could remember for sure – recreate the sensations of life in the womb. The rocking and gentle stretches, which are all part of this treatment, make you feel like a baby anyway!

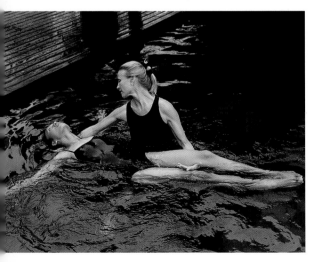

Thanks to the buoyancy of the water for support, the body relaxes in free float. This is the optimum state for carrying out bodywork according to the principles of shiatsu, the Japanese form of massage that concentrates on the body's meridians to stimulate its energy flow and de-stress. The mind goes into limbo as the body is walked very slowly around the pool and gently rocked. This is the starting point for various sequences that revolve, massage and outstretch the limbs. Ardent followers claim that the treatment helps them get in touch with deep feelings of safety and connectedness. However you choose to look at it, Water Shiatsu is – for sure – a total tune-out and the ultimate unwind! Try it at a *Breathing Space* weekend retreat or at their *Moana Spa*, both on the Indonesian island of Batam.

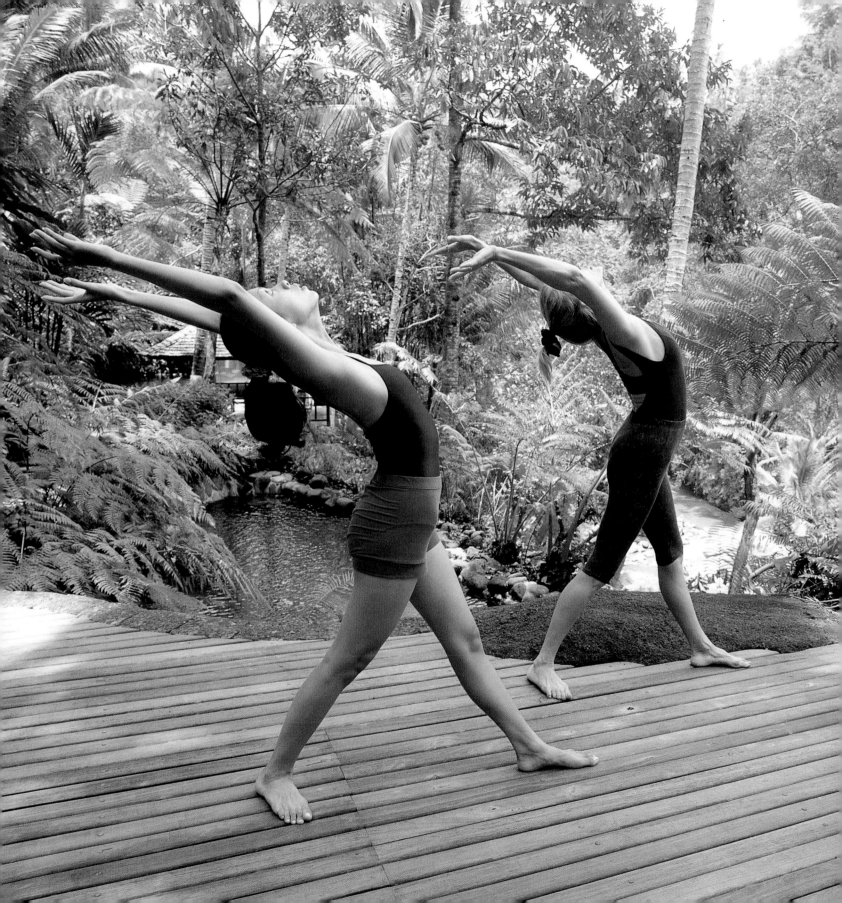

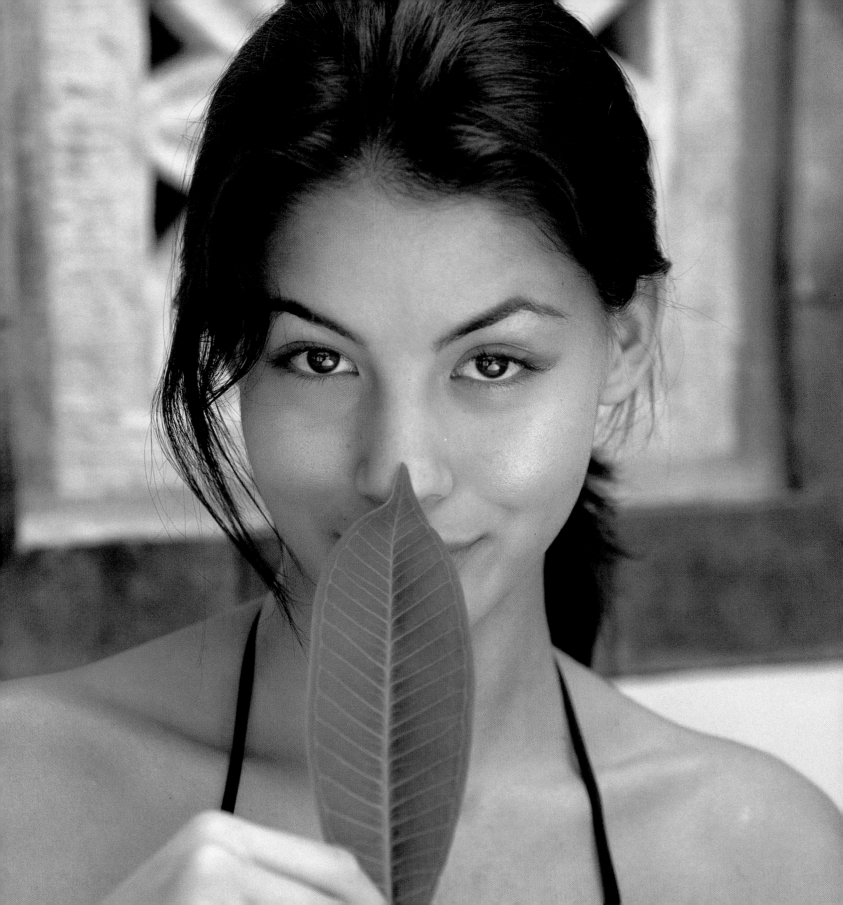

face value

More than any other part of our body, our face reflects most accurately what is going on beneath our skin's façade. It is the clearest indication of the popular maxim: 'beauty from the inside-out'. While we know that we cannot halt our natural ageing process, we can help our skins age with grace by taking a few simple steps. Fresh air, adequate sleep, a high water intake, relaxation and a diet high in fruit and vegetables and low in processed foods, all help our facial skin stay plump and relatively free from blemishes.

Tropical Asian women have a head start on those in the West. These basic steps have been an integral part of their traditional lifestyles for centuries. And many of their facial preparations are mixed directly from the vast botanical heritage that this region lays claim to. For example, many natural beauty preparations stem from the palaces in Central Java where princesses spent their youth learning and preparing them for their own use. In the absence of night creams, neck creams and new oxygen creams, Asian women have used raw plant extracts to slough off dead skin cells, fight acne, replenish moisture or achieve an SPF.

Now that 'natural' is *de rigueur* once more, women are flocking to Asian spas where traditional treatments, free from clinical input, are giving them soft skin and a relaxed state of mind. 'Back to basics' is the new concept for modern beauty, and ironically, they may now find themselves having their faces 'cleaned' with the very food that, at home, they have hastily wiped from their chins.

Traditional Honey-Cucumber Facial

The principle ingredients of this facial – honey, lime and cucumber – enjoy an age-old reputation as skin healers, softeners and moisturizers. Used in conjunction with each other, these three natural ingredients reduce the discomforts of skin irritations and stem infection while promoting new cell growth.

This simple and sensual facial, offered at *Banyan Tree Spa Bintan* and *Banyan Tree Spa Phuket*, leaves your skin feeling soft and plump and your mind questioning the need for progress in the beauty industry. Who needs electric steamers, electro-magnetic currents, alpha-hydroxy creams for wrinkle reduction and ultimately cosmetic surgery, when nature can be so gentle on the skin and so much kinder on the complexion? Scientific intervention is part of the skincare regimen of the past.

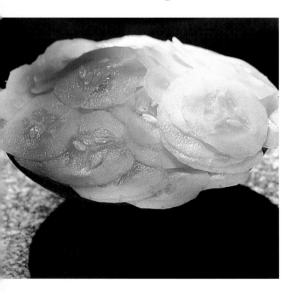

For Scrub

8 oz (1 cup)	clear honey (Thai honey is the most nutritious for this)
10 drops	fresh lime juice
1	medium-sized cucumber, thinly sliced

Steps

1. Cleanse your face with warm water and a natural cloth.
2. Mix the honey and lime juice together and massage into your face for 15 minutes. The sticky-turned-slippery sensation is sublime. The lime peels away surface cells and the honey softens the skin.
3. Wipe away the residue of honey with a wet, warm cloth. Pat dry.
4. Neatly place the cucumber patches over your face and neck (covering eyes and mouth is optional). They feel cool while they tighten the skin and replenish moisture.
5. Finishing with a delicate moisturizer is optional, but not necessary.

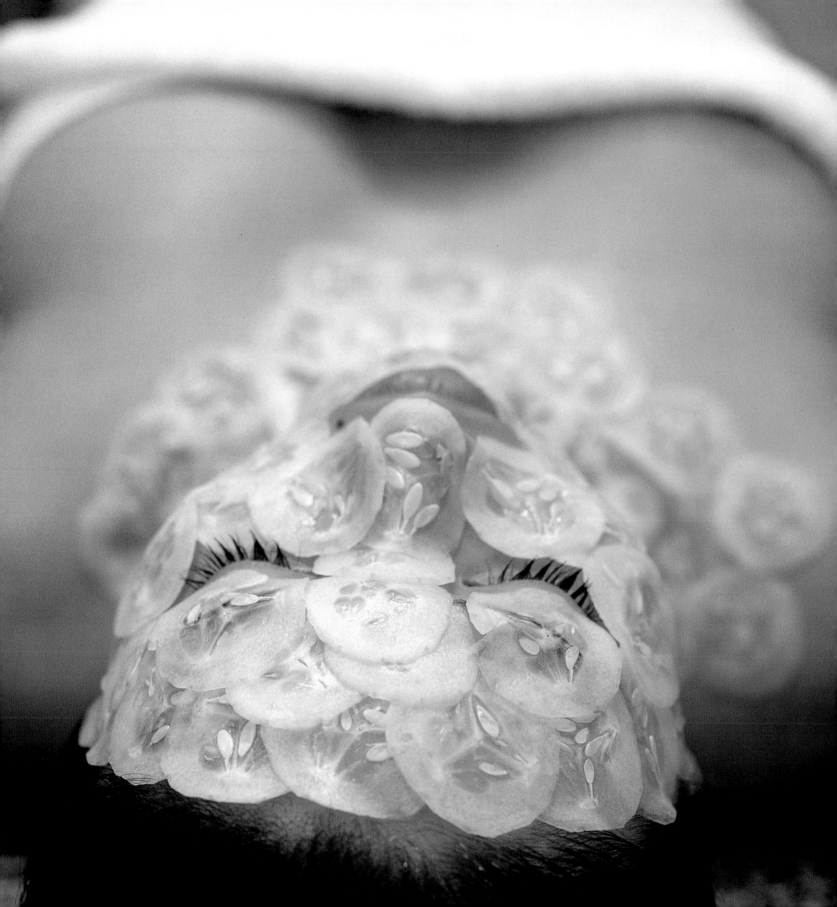

Kitchen Cosmetics

There are all sorts of things in the kitchen cabinets and fridge that can be used for a cleansing and refreshing facial. As part of their five-day Spa Indulgence programme, the *Mandara Spa at The Chedi* in Ubud, Bali, offers an afternoon of practical and fun experiments. Their Kitchen Cosmetics class can be done easily at home as a way of using up what you did not get round to eating. And don't forget that it's only with these sorts of fridge facials that you know *exactly* what you are putting on your skin.

The following can be done in sequence or separately. Word from the 'tried-and-tested' mouths is: "Do these once a month, your skin will feel totally new for three days and will never break out."

Lemon Refresher

Slightly astringent and tightening for the face

1	lemon or lime
1/2 tsp	cold water

Mix the lemon or lime juice and the water in a bowl. Gently pat on to your face after any of the treatments on right. The lemon/lime's acidity acts as a toner to tighten the skin and close the pores after a facial. It smells great too!

Egg White Mask

Tightening for a lacklustre complexion

1	egg

Break open the egg and separate the white from the yolk. Beat the white for one minute by hand. Gently apply to the skin and let it harden. Wash off with warm water. The egg white draws toxins from the skin's surface and tightens the pores as it cleans.

Honey Pat

Softening and lifting for the face

    2 tbsp   runny honey

    2 tsp   lime juice (optional)

Dip your fingers into a bowl containing the honey and lime juice and gently pat onto your skin. Using circular motions, rotate your fingers upward from your chin, cheeks and forehead. Change to a typing motion, tapping the skin and honey until it feels sticky. Let the honey sit for 15 minutes before rinsing off with warm water. Honey is effective in helping your skin to retain moisture.

Polenta and Yoghurt Scrub

Cleansing and exfoliating for face and body

    1 tbsp   ground corn meal (polenta)

    2 tbsp   natural yoghurt

Mix into a paste and gently rub into your skin, starting at the chin and working up to the cheeks and forehead in small circles. The exfoliating properties of the corn's gritty texture leave your face invigorated and glowing.

Avocado Mask

Softening and nourishing for face and body

    1   avocado

Mash the creamy insides into a soft paste and apply to your face using the avocado stone to massage the flesh into your skin with small, upward, circular motions. Wash off with warm water after a few minutes. The nourishing oil is naturally rich in vitamin E and leaves your skin feeling soft.

Traditional Facial

While the concept of the Western facial and its ritual process of toning and scrubbing has no roots in tropical Asian culture, one bumper spa facial combines fresh-from-the-garden produce with some natural skincare products manufactured in Indonesia. This Traditional Facial, found at all Mandara Spas (at *The Chedi, Ibah, Bali Padma* and *Nikko* in Bali, *Novotel* in Lombok and Malaysia's *The Datai*), includes massage as an unexpected added bonus.

For Scrub

15 gm (1 tbsp)	dry corn kernel
15 gm (1 tbsp)	ground rice powder
15 ml (1 tbsp)	cucumber juice (for oily skin)
or	
15 ml (1 tbsp)	carrot juice (for normal/dry skin)

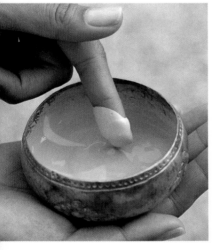

For Mask

20 gm (2 tbsp)	collagen powder (or cosmetic clay powder available at health shops)
10 ml (1 tbsp)	cucumber juice (for oily skin)
or	
10 ml (1 tbsp)	carrot juice (for normal/dry skin)
2	cucumber slices for eyes

For Toning and Moisturizing

Martha Tilaar's *Biokos* cleanser, toner and moisturizer with a seaweed base (*see page 175*)

Steps

1   Mix the corn (dried, yellow kernels) together with the rice powder (finely ground rice). Then add the cucumber or carrot juice to make your scrub.

2   After your cleansing and toning routine (Mandara Spas use the seaweed-rich line *Biokos*, from Martha Tilaar), apply the scrub, taking care not to rub too vigorously as over-zealous rubbing can do more harm than good. Concentrate on the nose area.

3   (While this scrub settles, massage your feet and calves with your favourite oil.)

4   Gently wipe off the scrub, ideally with a natural sponge or muslin cloth dipped in warm water. Tone and moisturize with Martha Tilaar's *Biokos* toner and moisturizer with a seaweed base.

5   Mix the collagen powder (or the cosmetic clay powder, depending on which you use) together with the cucumber or carrot juice to make the mask.

6   Apply the mask with your fingers or a brush and place the cucumber patches over your eyes. (This is where you need a friend who will massage your hands and arms while you drift off under the cooling and tightening mask.)

7   After 15 minutes, gently wipe off the mask with a natural sponge or muslin cloth dipped in warm water.

8   Tone and moisturize and, while massaging the face, skip your fingers over your forehead and cheeks to stimulate your nerve endings.

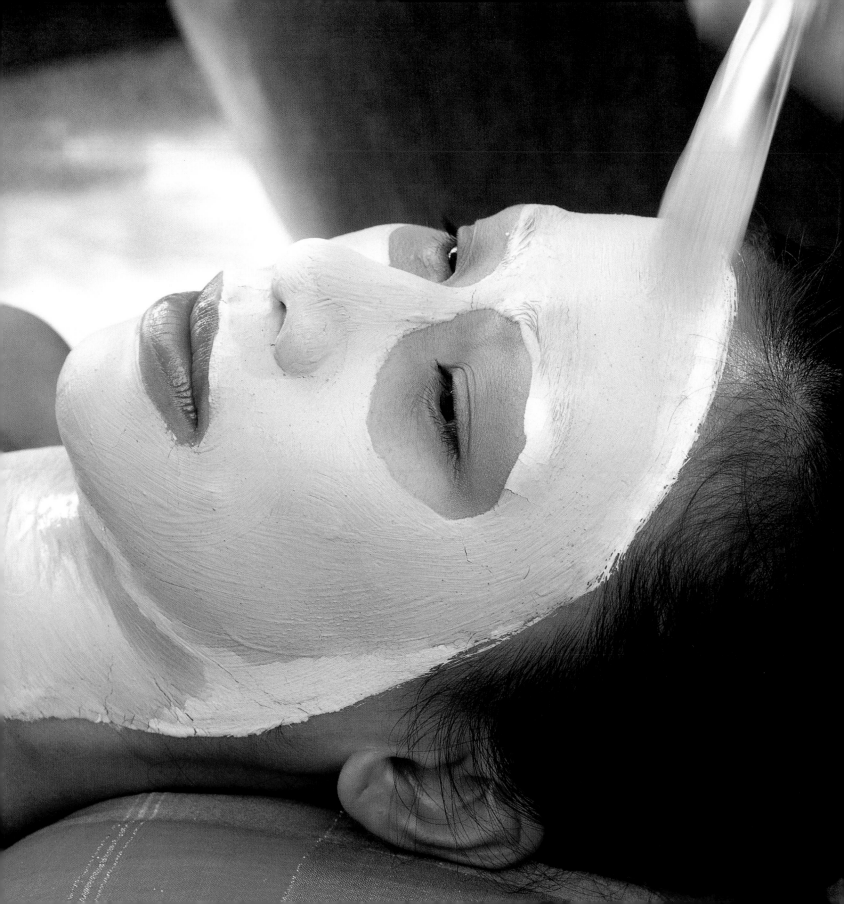

Jamu Tropical Nuts Facial

This facial is fresh from the Indonesian market place and good enough to eat: marzipan scents, cucumber, nuts, lemon grass and warm, melting honey. It was designed especially for *Jamu Body Treatments* in Jakarta according to traditional folklore relating to the medicinal and beautifying agents of local produce. Before doing this facial, prepare the following:

Cucumber Toner

1	small cucumber with skin but not seeds

Blend for 30 seconds. Strain the juice as a toner, but store both the juice and the flesh separately in a fridge.

Almond Milk

20 gms (2 tbsp)	clean, skinned almonds
50 mls ($^{1}/_{2}$ cup)	water

Whiz both in a blender until smooth, about two minutes. Strain several times through a fine mesh cheesecloth to obtain almond milk. Store both the milk and the almond meat in separate containers in the fridge.

City Grime Cleanser

2 tsp	olive oil
1 tsp	thick or runny honey

Mix together.

Kemiri Nut (Candlenut) Milk

For Kemiri Nut Scrub, on right

20 gms (2 tbsp)	*kemiri* nuts
50 mls ($^{1}/_{2}$ cup)	water

Whiz both in a blender until smooth, about two minutes. Strain the mixture several times through a fine mesh cheesecloth until the *kemiri* milk is a silky consistency. Store both the milk and the *kemiri* nut meat in separate containers in the fridge.

Lemon Grass Infusion

For Kemiri Nut Scrub, on right

250 gms ($^{1}/_{2}$ lb)	lemon grass
250 gms (2 cups)	boiling water

Pour the boiling water over the lemon grass. Cover the container and let it stand for 20 minutes until the liquid has cooled down. Strain.

Kemiri Nut (Candlenut) Scrub

10 gms (1 tbsp)	*kemiri* nut meat
1 tsp	*kemiri* nut milk
1 tsp	Lemon Grass Infusion (*see left*)

Mix together into a moist paste. Mix in the Lemon Grass Infusion until the consistency feels right for you.

Almond, Oatmeal and Cucumber Mask

For oily or problem skin

5 cm (2 inches)	unpeeled cucumber
1 tbsp	Almond Milk (*see left*)
40 gms (4 tbsp)	rolled oats
1–2 tbsp	kaolin powder

If you are making this mask separately from the rest of these facial ingredients, blend the cucumber for about 30 seconds, then gently strain the liquid away from the pulp. If you have already made the Cucumber Toner, use the pulp that you have saved from this. Mix all the ingredients together well. Add only enough kaolin powder to make a paste that is dry but workable. The more kaolin used, the faster the mask will dry and the more it will feel tight on your skin.

Avocado, Coconut, Almond and Cucumber Mask

For dry, sun-damaged or ageing skin

5 cm (2 inches)	unpeeled cucumber
1 tbsp	Almond Milk (*see left*)
1/4 fruit	avocado flesh
2 tbsp	coconut oil (or other vegetable oil)
2–3 tbsp	kaolin powder

If you are making this mask separately from the rest of these facial ingredients, blend the cucumber for about 30 seconds, then gently strain the liquid away from the pulp. If you have already made the Cucumber Toner, use the pulp that you have saved from this. Mix all the ingredients together well. Add only enough kaolin powder to make a paste that is dry but workable. The more kaolin used, the faster the mask will dry and the more it will feel tight on your skin.

Steps

1. Clean away any make-up using Cucumber Toner or Almond Milk.
2. Using quick, circular strokes, briskly massage the City Grime Cleanser into the face and neck, concentrating on problem areas.
3. Steam your face and neck with a warm, wet towel and wipe it clean.
4. Apply the Kemiri Nut Scrub to your face using brisk, circular but gentle movements.
5. Wipe off the scrub using a hot, wet towel.
6. Massage your face (and neck and ears) with the Almond Milk. Using your fingers, massage from chin to cheeks to nose to forehead to temples to ears.
7. Steam your face with a hot, wet, towel and wipe away any excess Almond Milk.
8. Cleanse and tone your face with the Cucumber Toner.
9. Apply either the Almond, Oatmeal and Cucumber Mask or the Avocado, Coconut, Almond and Cucumber Mask, depending on your skin type, on both face and neck with a small brush. Leave it for 15–20 minutes.
10. Wipe off the mask using a hot, wet towel and then lay an ice-cold towel on your face. Blot with a tissue.
11. Finish by applying some Cucumber Toner and Almond Milk to re-hydrate the skin.

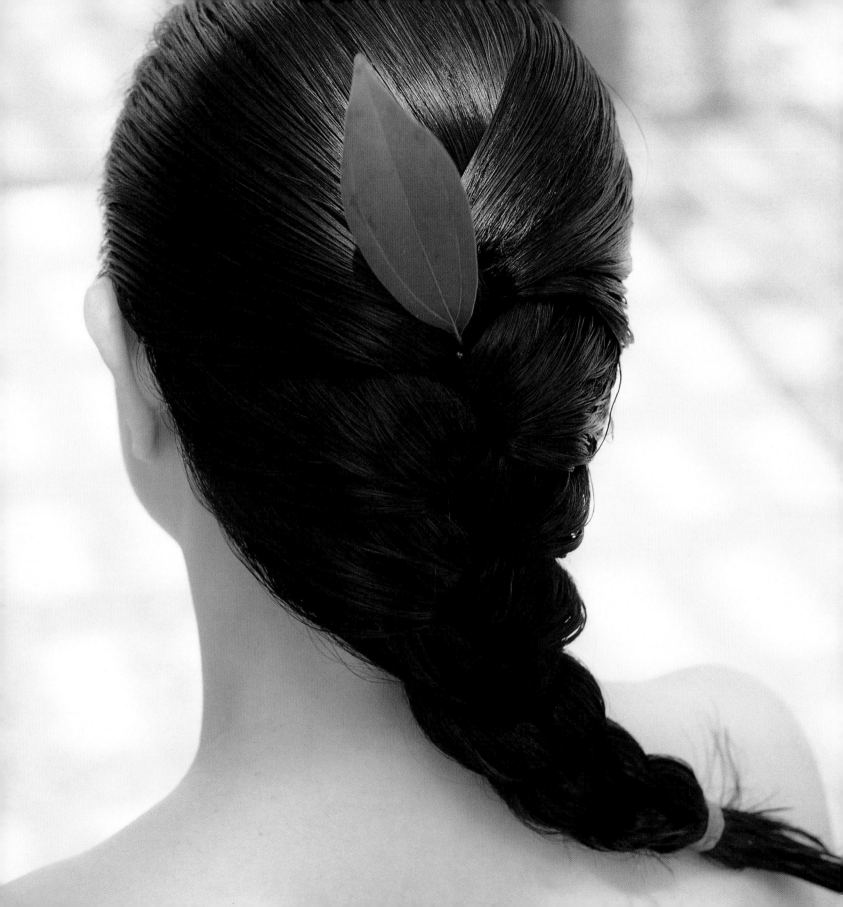

hair story

There is so much truth in the old cliché of 'having a bad hair day'. Feeling bad about the cut, style, touch, bounce and shimmer of our hair – or, more precisely, the lack of these – affects our morale like nothing else. But just like our skin, our hair is a barometer of our general health; it becomes duller and lankier the more tired and poorly nourished we are. It needs fresh air, fresh foods, sleep and low stress levels to maintain its shine. It also depends on a healthy scalp; a good scalp massage activates hair follicles and reduces tension in our heads.

One of the most striking features of tropical Asian women's beauty is their sleek and shiny hair. Historically their locks have been so lustrous precisely because of the lack of detergents available to them and their con-sequent reliance on nature's yield. Today, shampoo has taken over from coconut oil for washing, but hair remains a major focus of beauty ritual, and all manner of natural produce – flowers, oils, plant matter – are regularly applied to keep it glossy. Added to this, the traditional Asian diet based on fruit, vegetables, whole grains and oily fish is perfect nourishment for healthy hair.

While proper cleaning and conditioning provides some of the best protection from environmental attack, manufactured hair products that contain harsh stripping chemicals can do more harm than good. This chapter highlights some more natural remedies, tried and tested by the very women who tout those thick black tresses that speak for themselves.

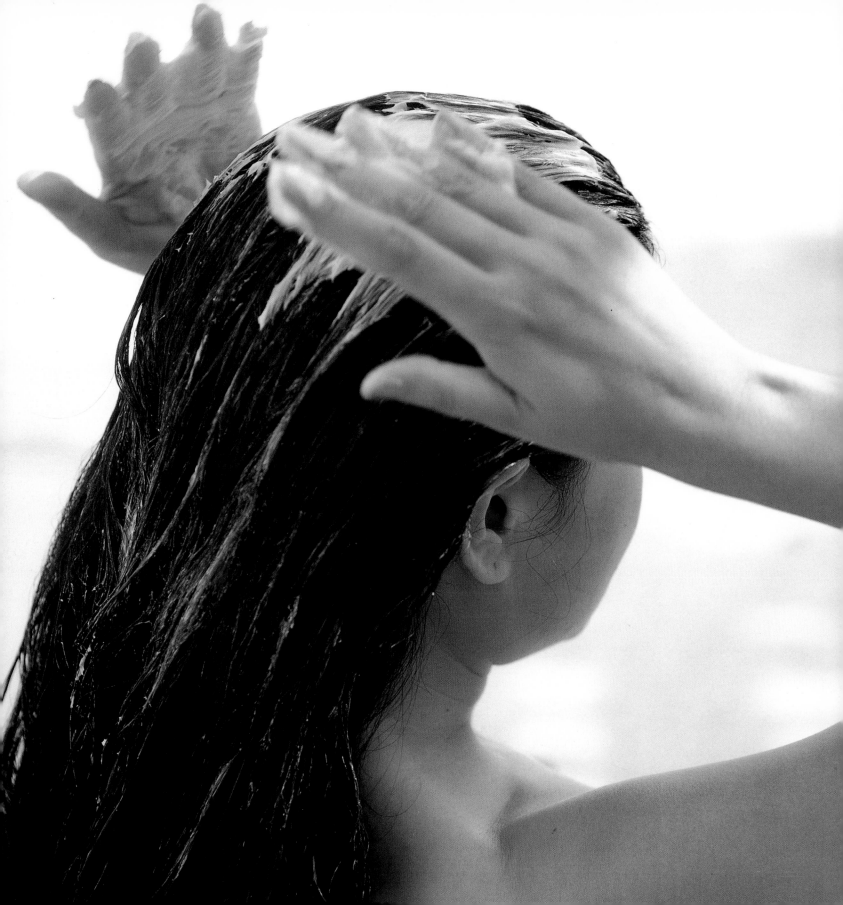

Crème Bath Hair Treatment

The crème bath is synonymous with hair salons everywhere in Asia where hair is a major focus of beauty ritual. It is one of the most popular methods of maintaining the sleek and shiny texture for which Asian women's hair is renowned.

Although often referred to as a 'traditional' head treatment, the crème bath is based on a manufactured product, namely a rich conditioning cream, whose thick glutinous consistency thoroughly coats the hair like icing. After steaming, it is washed off to leave hair superlatively soft and shiny.

Natural ingredients are often added to the crème bath product to treat specific hair conditions. The *St Gregory Javana Spa* in Singapore offers Indonesian-produced hair crèmes for specific hair types for their 90-minute *Mandi Kepala*.

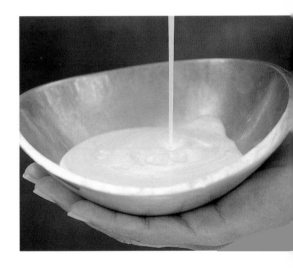

The therapists run their crème-coated fingers through section after section of hair leaving your head feeling cool, clammy, heavy and 'gooey'. Then lie back to the touch of rhythmic finger movements that massage the scalp and gradually move down the neck and shoulders. While you drift off into limbo, the crème is stimulating the scalp and the hair follicles and softening and strengthening the strands of hair.

Natural Crème Bath Additives

Here are some of the flavours recommended for specific hair conditions:

Carrot	for hair growth
Henna	for nourishing dry or permed hair
Avocado	for feeding dry hair
Ginseng	for strengthening the hair roots
Celery	for increasing hair elasticity
Aloe vera	for a general hair food
Candlenut	for promoting glossy, dark hair
Seaweed	for stimulating hair growth
Egg	for healing dry hair and split ends

Aromatherapy Scalp Treatment

This treatment, found exclusively at the *Spa at Bali Hyatt*, Sanur, Bali, must rank among the best head remedies available anywhere. It incorporates a crème bath but also makes use of gels, oils and a heaven-sent massage to awaken your brain, stimulate hair growth and relax the body.

Ingredients

10 mls (1 tbsp)	hot macadamia oil
5 mls (½ tsp)	essential oil of your choice
3 tbsp	manufactured crème bath

Steps

1 Warm the macadamia oil in an aromatherapy oil burner with your choice of essential oils which are the active ingredients of this treatment (see below). The ratio between base and essential oils should be 2:1. Macadamia oil is used because, unlike the traditional coconut oil, it does not have an aroma that interferes with the scent of the essential oils. The oil is heated so that it penetrates the hair more easily.

2 With your fingers, part the hair. Using a face mask applicator brush, smear the warm oil along the scalp line at one-inch intervals massaging with your finger tips as you go.

3 When your scalp is fairly well covered with oil apply the crème bath from the roots to the ends of your hair and massage your scalp with finger tip pressure. Snap sections of your scalp between fingers and thumb for added stimulation.

4 For best results, cover your head with a loose, clear shower cap and steam for 10–20 minutes, or leave for 20 minutes.

5 Shampoo several times to remove all traces of oil.

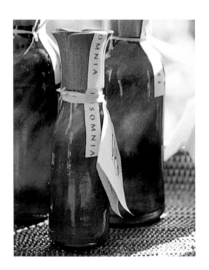

Essential Oils

Best essential oils for the hair as recommended by the *Spa at Bali Hyatt*.

Dry hair	geranium, sandalwood, palmarosa, lavender
Damaged hair	geranium, lavender, sandalwood, frankincense
Blond hair	geranium, lemon, camomile
Grey hair	camomile, sage, lavender, rose
Hair loss	juniper, rosemary, lavender
Dandruff/excema	eucalyptus, rosemary, cedarwood, tea tree

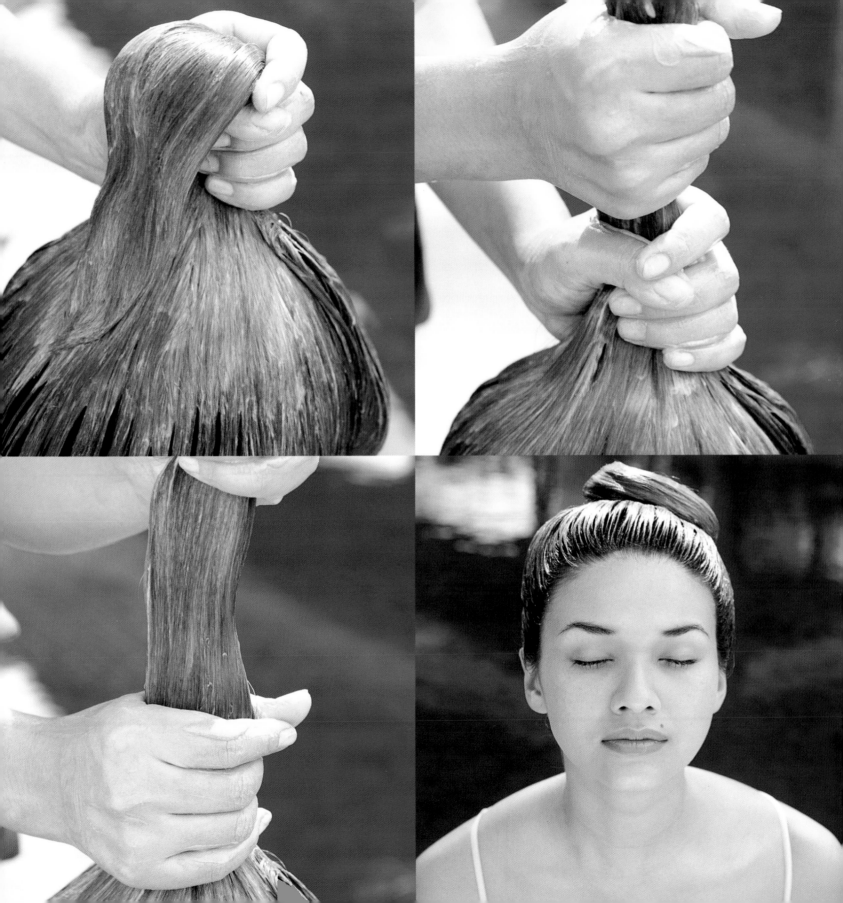

Hibiscus Hair Shampoo

The leaves from the prolific hibiscus bush *(waru)* were commonly used for hair washing in Indonesia before the advent of manufactured shampoo. When mashed these leaves excrete a sticky gel, similar to aloe vera.

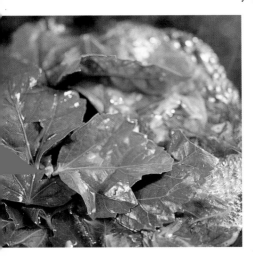

Ingredients

large handful	hibiscus leaves
to cover	water

Steps

1. Crush the leaves loosely in your hand and barely cover them with water. Boil for 20 minutes. Strain.
2. The remaining liquid has a sticky, gel-like consistency which forms a lather when massaged into the head.
3. Rinse.

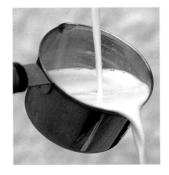

Coconut Milk

Young girls say their grandmothers still wash their hair with coconut milk. They use thick milk for washing and massaging, lighter milk from a younger coconut for conditioning and rinsing. But for most, this is considered crazily old fashioned and far too much like hard work! It's worth a try though.

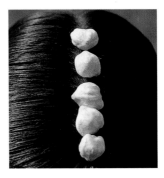

Nuts for Hair

Loosely grind a handful of rich candlenuts (*kemiri* nuts) until their oil starts to seep out. Pan fry them briefly. As they turn brown and their nutty aroma is released, smash them again. Massage the nut and the oil into the scalp and leave for 15 minutes. Myth has it that your hair will resist turning grey. Candlenuts also leave your hair super-shiny.

Merang Hair Treatment

In the wonderful world of nature, beauty picks up where agriculture leaves off: watermelon rinds and papaya skins, for example, do a great turn as a face mask before being consigned to the bin. Another great example where beauty thrives off nature's cast-offs is redundant rice crops (*merang*) which keep grey hair at bay. The *merang* head treatment has been practised throughout tropical Asia for centuries.

The only spa offering *merang* is the *Spa at Hotel Tugu*, Bali. In fact, this spa offers the most comprehensive range of such real, rural remedies.

Ingredients

one handful	*merang* – burnt rice paddy stalks
one small bowl	water

Steps

1 Soak the burnt rice stalks in the water overnight so that the ash comes loose and dissolves. Strain several times and keep the water.

2 Pour this inky liquid onto the head and rub into the scalp. Watch it foam like shampoo. The liquid has cleansing properties and acts as a tonic.

3 Your head will feel tingly and your hair soft and clean. Any grey hairs will be dyed a darker shade. Although you do not need to have black hair for this treatment, blondes should not experiment! Locals claim that this treatment is most effective when regularly applied.

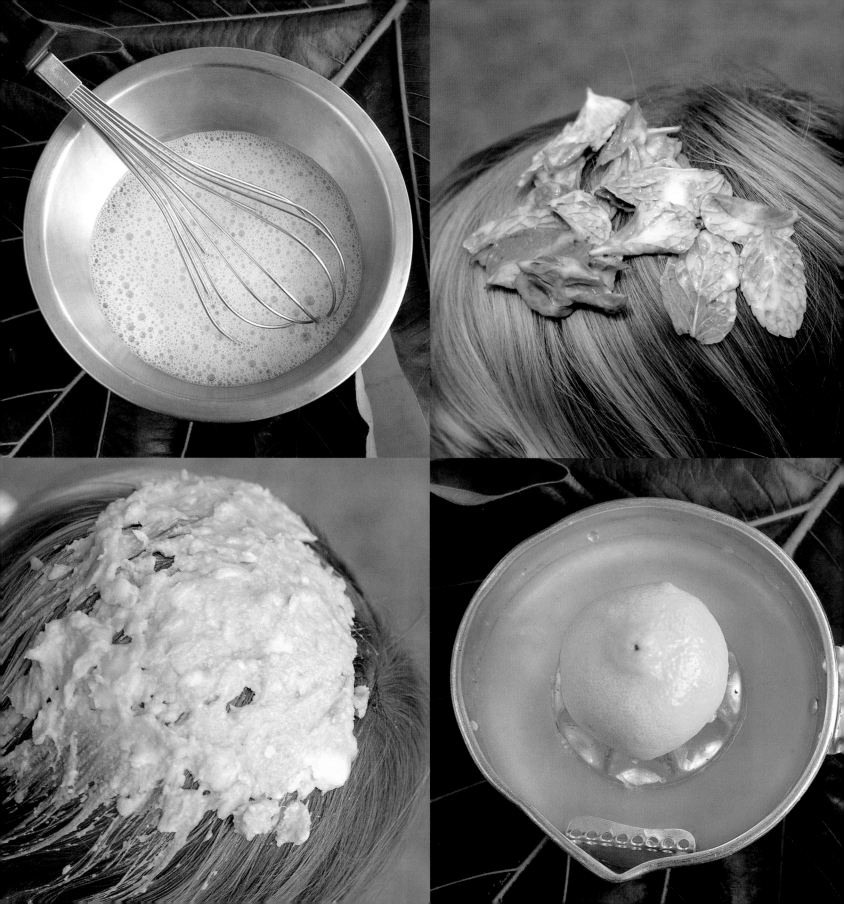

Hair Remedies

For Dry Hair
- Massage the creamy insides of an avocado into clean dry hair and leave for 15–20 minutes.
- Massage coconut oil into your hair and leave for a few hours. Wash several times before your hair feels silky rather than oily.

For Lacklustre Hair
- Massage two large, grated carrots into damp or dry hair. Trap with a bath hat and leave for 15–20 minutes.
- Squeeze half a lemon into 200 mls (1 cup) of water and use the mixture as a final rinse after shampooing.

For Thinning Hair
- Whisk two eggs and massage them into your hair. Wash off after ten minutes to enhance hair growth and strength.
- Put several sticks of celery through a juicer and massage the juice into your scalp. Leave for 15 minutes before washing.

For Dandruff
- Mix a large handful of crushed mint leaves into your conditioner and leave on the hair for 15–20 minutes.

For Fragrant Hair
The sweet-smelling jasmine bud plays an important role in beauty ritual throughout Asia. In Thailand and Indonesia the small flowers are woven into a bride's hair on her wedding day. This type of head-dressing continues among married women in the palaces of Central Java while unmarried women, according to palace tradition, should weave their hair with the fragrant pandanus leaf avoiding any form of flower until she is wed.

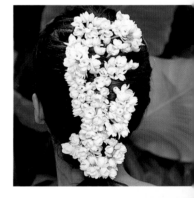

Embrace the exotic and try pinning a few jasmine blooms into your hair as much for the sweet scent as the pretty effect. It is best to plait the hair, thread a classic hairpin through the base of the flower and then wedge the pin into the thick plait of hair.

For Thicker Hair
Aloe vera plants, known in Indonesia as 'alligator's tongue' because of their spiky appearance, grow wild throughout tropical Asia. Their thick spiny leaves contain a cooling sap, which is an elixir for heavy heads. More precisely this extract contains a natural tannin with an anti-inflammatory effect, and saponin, a natural emulsifier.

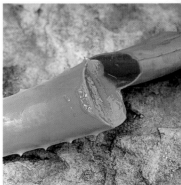

- Break open an aloe vera leaf with a knife to reveal a sticky juice. Massage the juice into the scalp and leave it for 15 minutes. Wash off.
- Feel your scalp cool down and tingle. The aloe's active ingredients stimulate the follicles for a thick and fuller head of hair.

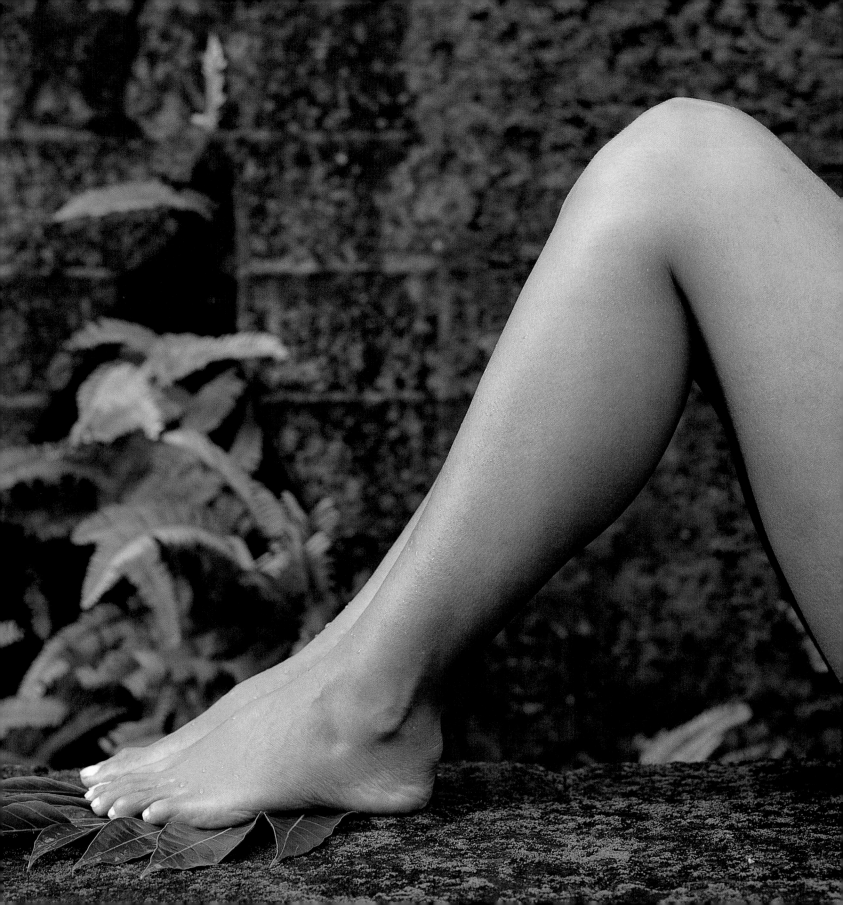

feet first

Of all our body parts, our feet tend to suffer most. They are our trusty servants, yet we stuff them into shoes and pay little respect to the fact that they carry our whole body weight. During our lifetime, they traipse four times around the world or roughly 70,000 miles. In cold weather we ignore them as they are under wraps; when it is hot we pay them scant attention with a swoosh of nail varnish before displaying them in sandals. And we wonder why 'our feet are killing us' as that painful saying goes. There's nothing worse than sore feet, but it is a guaranteed condition if we don't look after them.

Yet our own two feet are crucial in helping us to look after our bodies just by walking. Walking tones our heart and lungs and so boosts our energy. It lowers cholesterol levels, burns calories and therefore helps us to lose weight. Medics also claim that walking reduces the risk of developing osteoporosis, which makes older bones brittle and prone to fracture.

Needless to say, in Asia an ancient technique for foot relief has been practised for centuries. It originated in India and China more than 5,000 years ago and is known loosely as reflexology. It has grown out of the understanding that every part of our faithful pair of feet corresponds to a part of our body, making them key healing zones.

After all, one quarter of all our body's bones (26 different bones) are resident in our feet. It seems they deserve as much, if not more, attention than any other part of our body.

How to...happy feet

Happy feet make happy people. Remember that anointing the feet is a long-held ritual in many cultures. As you rub on these ointments think that you are giving a sacred start – or finish – to your day. This is an almost religious act of gratitude for your mobility! Here are some quick and easy ways to cheer all three of you up.

Pedicure

A pedicure is not simply the pursuit of vanity. A proper one should include a foot soak, a nail trim, which prevents in-growing toenails, and the removal of hard skin and calluses which could, if left, lead to corns. Cuticles should be pushed down, not cut, and feet and calves massaged with cream or oil if skin is particularly dry. An olive oil base is especially nourishing. Painted nails look shiniest and last longest if they get a clear undercoat, two coats of colour and a clear top coat. Polish takes at least 15 minutes to dry.

Most major spas offer a full-on pedicure, although some therapists are more professional than others who can take far too long and poke about in tender spots, so be wary.

Hard Skin

One of the most effective exfoliants for hard skin that develops on the soles of the feet is sand. Collect some ordinary beach sand on your next visit to a tropical spa and mix it with enough vegetable oil to make a sticky paste. Add a few drops of peppermint or rosemary essential oil to complete the invigorating experience. Massage your feet concentrating on the heels, the balls and the big toes where skin is usually hardest.

Quick Tips
1. Cool down hot feet with a peppermint and aloe vera gel rub.
2. Soothe tired feet with a vegetable oil massage spiked with clove oil which has anesthetic properties. Best base oils for feet include avocado, olive and sesame.
3. Soak your feet in warm water laced with pine, tea tree and eucalyptus oils to banish odours.
4. Exercise and strengthen your foot muscles by rolling each foot over a tennis ball while sitting down.
5. Detoxify your whole body with a 10-minute foot soak in warm water containing two tablespoons of rock salt. Follow with an oil massage.
6. Avoid bunions and ankle problems and ditch your high heels. If impossible, wear them sparingly! Keep infections away and change your tights and socks every day. Make sure they, like your shoes, are never too small. Let your feet breathe whenever you can.

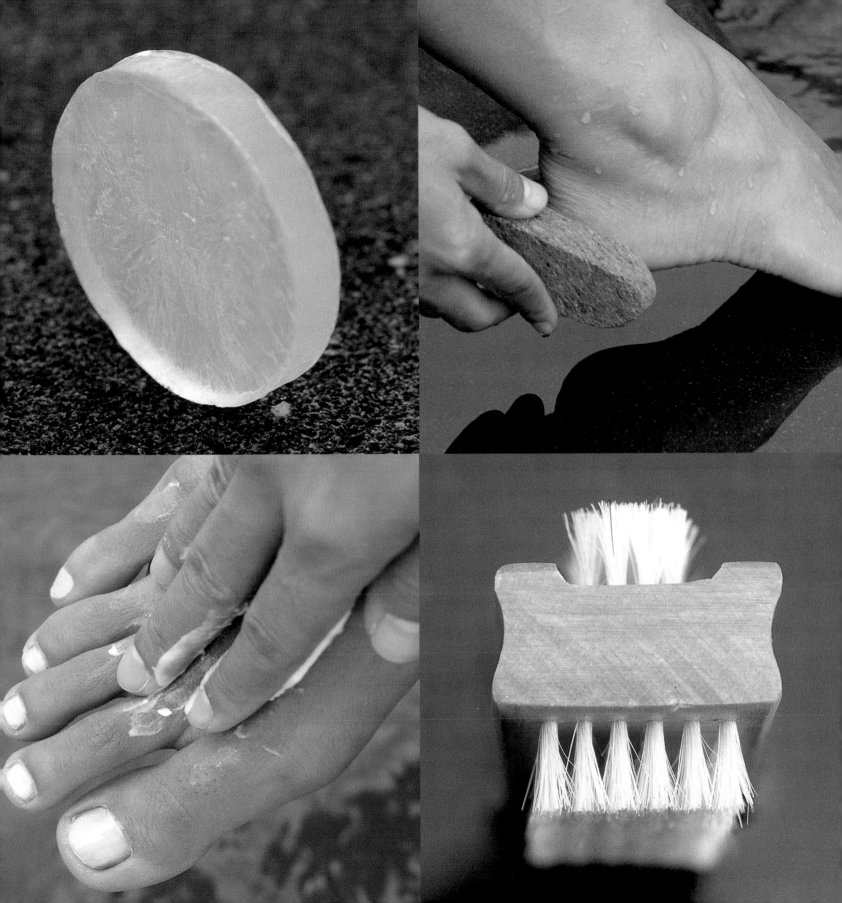

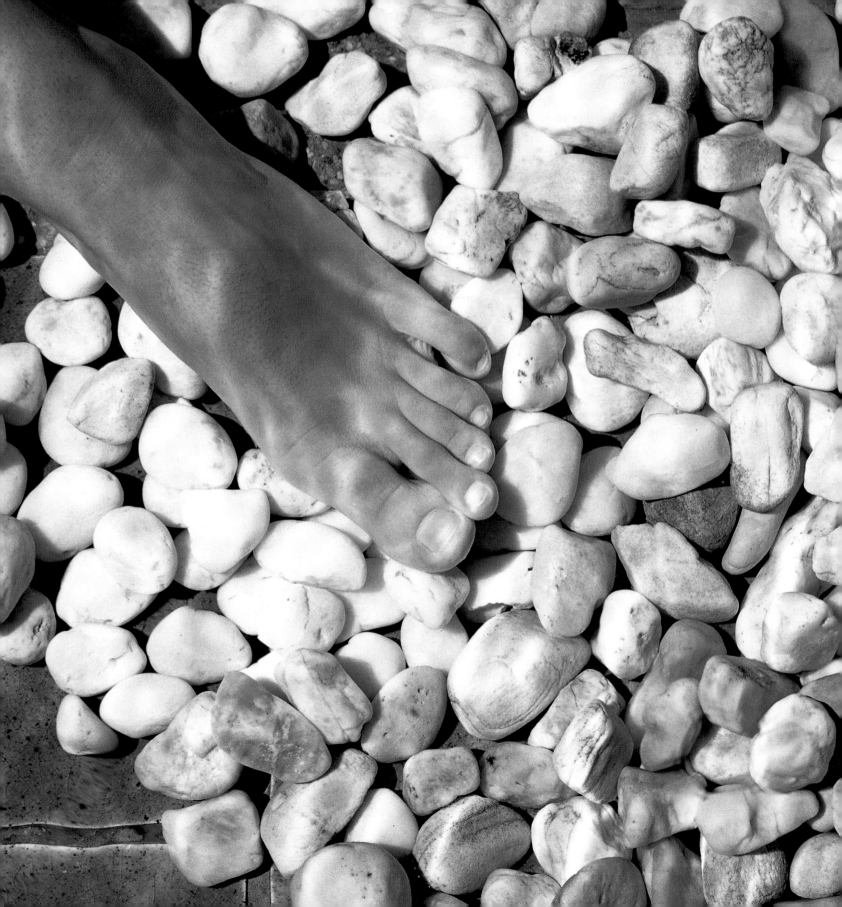

Kneipp Foot Bath

This is a one-off experience on the Asian spa circuit, exclusive to Thailand's *Chiva-Som*. The foot bath itself comprises a corridor, calf-deep with water floating on a bed of stones. The water is cold, the corridor dark and the sensation exhilarating if a little painful on your soles. While it's a relief to step out of the bumpy foot bath onto a flat, dry surface, your feet tingle and your whole body feels alive. You are compelled to walk another circuit, for kicks!

This bath is based on the theory of a 19th-century Bavarian priest, Father Sebastian Kneipp. He systemized the healing properties of water into the science of hydrotherapy and was famous for preaching the health benefits of walking barefoot on dewy morning grass, in keeping with his belief that nature provides us with everything we need to be healthy and happy. At *Chiva-Som*, the foot bath combines the healing powers of water with the principle of reflexology, whereby the sensitive nerve endings in our feet are invigorated by the pressure of the small stones and the cold water.

As a consolation for the wincing you will do, this foot bath encircles *Chiva-Som*'s steam bath. Come out of the cold and step into this smoky hot chamber for more body blitzing!

Oriental Foot Massage

Oriental foot massage, otherwise known as reflexology or previously as zone therapy, is an ancient art of healing which works on the principle that the body's organs, including the brain, are connected by energy channels to trigger points in our feet. Consequently, when our feet are tired, so are our minds and bodies.

Reflexologists believe that if a body part (liver, thyroid, gall bladder, eyes and ears) is not functioning properly, the energy flowing through our channels, or meridians, becomes sluggish, even blocked. This can cause crystals to gather under the skin in specific parts of our feet. Massaging these points breaks down the crystals and restores the flow of body energy.

There are reputedly 7,000 nerve endings in our feet and therapists know which area mirrors which body part. Asians are particularly intuitive when it comes to massaging feet and a treatment of this ilk is offered in most spas, either alone or as part of other massage therapies. It is fabulous for stimulating circulation and restoring physical and mental harmony. It is also an uncannily accurate way of both detecting and healing internal problems.

Foot and Nut Treatment

The felons for corns and carbuncles are fashion footwear, tights and high heels, all of which we thrust upon our faithful feet. Give them time out and treat them to a weekly foot soak and massage, but if you find yourself in Bali, do not leave until your trotters have tried this bumper foot treatment at *Jamu Traditional Spa*, Kuta. They never knew life could be so good. If you are doing this Foot and Nut Treatment at home, prepare the following before starting:

Honey Milk Cleansing Lotion

10 pieces	*kemiri* nut (candlenut)
3 tbsp	honey
4 tbsp	water

Blend the *kemiri* nuts and water together for two minutes. Using a fine mesh cheesecloth strain the milk from the meat. Save the meat for the Kemiri Nut Scrub and two tablespoons of the milk for the flower mask. Add the honey to the milk and mix well. This is now ready to use.

Lemon Grass Infusion

For Kemiri Nut Scrub, on right

250 gms (¹/₂ lb)	lemon grass
250 gms (2 cups)	boiling water

Pour the boiling water over the lemon grass. Cover the container and let it stand for 20 minutes until the liquid has cooled down. Strain.

Kemiri Nut Scrub

as saved	*kemiri* nut meat
500 gms (2 cups)	Lemon Grass Infusion

Use the nut meat already prepared for the cleansing lotion and mix it with enough of the Lemon Grass Infusion to make a moist paste that can be sensually rubbed into your feet.

Flower Mask

5 tbsp	kaolin powder
2 tbsp	*kemiri* nut milk
1 tsp	ground cinnamon
1 tsp	ground cloves
1 tsp	ground ginger
handful	pandanus leaves, hibiscus, frangipani or other delicate flowers such as rose, finely chopped
5 drops	lavender essential oil

Mix all of these ingredients together into a paste that is dry but workable. The more kaolin used the faster the mask will dry and the cooler it will feel on your feet.

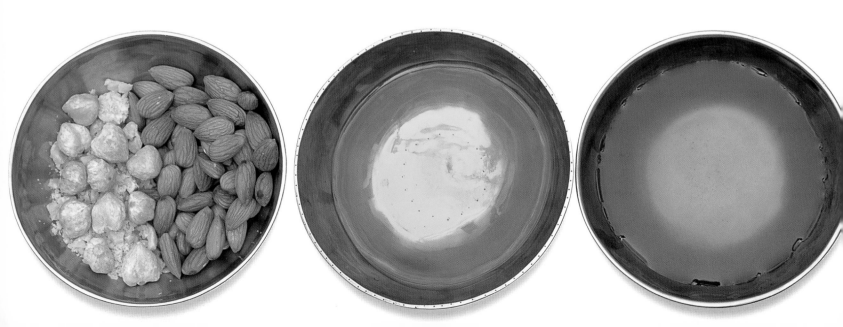

Steps

1   Wash your feet in a tub with a few drops of your favourite essential oil. Make sure you dry them properly between the toes and outwards along the nail growth on the side of each toe, removing all moisture so as to avoid infection.

2   Using cotton wool, rub the Honey Milk Cleansing Lotion all over each foot. The nut content is both astringent and deeply moisturizing while the honey both exfoliates some of the finer dead skin and softens it.

3   Relish rubbing your feet with the Kemiri Nut Scrub trapping the grains between your thumb and the nerve endings in the soles of your feet – there are over 7,000 of them! This very sensuous step leaves your feet wide awake and tingling.

4   Wipe away the scrub with a warm cloth and remove the finer traces with some more Honey Milk Cleansing Lotion.

5   Scoop the Flower Mask into the palm of your hands and pat it around your feet, covering them entirely up to the ankle to make two clay booties. It is best to sit back with your feet up on a stool covered with a towel. Enjoy the tightening and cooling sensation. Leave for 20 minutes before washing off with warm water.

6   Finish off with a calming aromatic foot massage using a rich carrier oil such as avocado, sesame or olive, plus a few drops of your favourite essential oil.

This is quite a labour-intensive treatment if done at home, but leaves your feet feeling loose and fluid. It is altogether a more divine experience at *Jamu Traditional Spa* where you sit back under the dappled shade of a banyan tree. Here therapists treat your calves as well as your feet. Both are cosseted for an hour and a half.

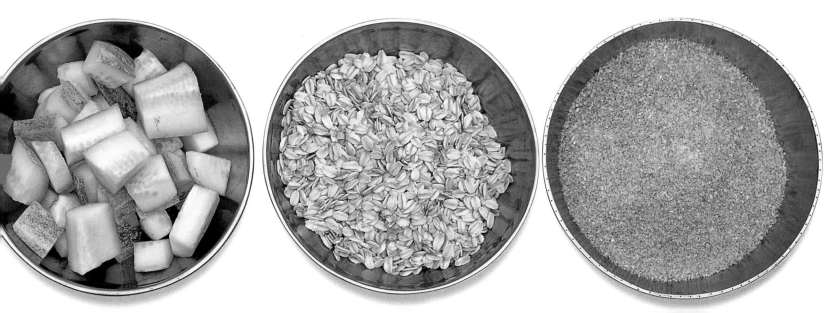

Floral Foot Soak

Soaking feet in warm water is an ancient form of pain relief practised, in varying guises, throughout many cultures. For centuries people have dissolved Epsom salts to reduce swelling, rock salt to detoxify the whole body at bedtime, or peppermint oil to cool and tickle the nerve endings.

In Bali, the higher castes allegedly keep a bowl of water in the corner of their bedroom, filled with flowers and the oil of eucalyptus for a ritual cleansing at the end of the day. Foot washing is also a symbolic part of one of the many rites of passage in Balinese Hinduism, carried out as a sign of deference to Sang Hyang Widhi, one of the gods responsible for the order of balance and imbalance in our lives.

You can experience the most heavenly foot soak in Bali at the *Spa at Bali Hyatt* where it is given as a matter of course before every treatment. You don't even have to lift your foot in or out of the thick wooden tub!

The treatment consists of gentle splashing with the scented flower water and gentle skin sloughing with volcanic stone: soft, white stone for women and a coarser black one for men. After this, heavy feet shed tension and start floating. After patting them dry, your therapist will massage your feet and legs with oil, working up toward the heart, using her thumb and forefinger to apply pressure up the back of the calf from the ankle. According to massage theory these strokes relieve poor circulation, fluid retention and bladder problems. The whole experience is so pleasurable and focused (and it could never last long enough!) that it hardly matters what, if any, medical benefits are taking place.

Use essential oils in your own foot soak. The *Spa at Bali Hyatt* favours three drops each of thyme, vetiver and sage as a good combination to make skin smooth. Flowers are added as a symbolic gesture to wash away bad luck. As an intrinsic part of every day life in Asia, flowers represent a bridge to the natural world, taking on a spiritual and cleansing significance. Don't make the water too hot and soak for 10–15 minutes for best results. Follow by massaging your feet with a rich oil such as coconut, olive or avocado.

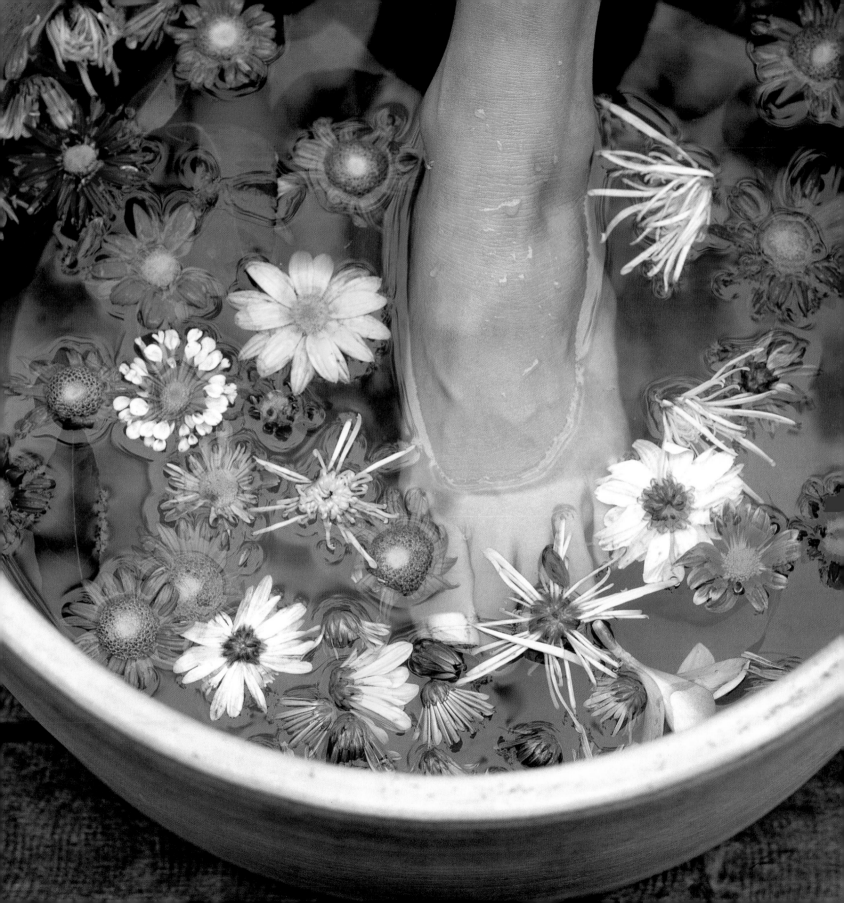

asian spa
cuisine

We have all heard the maxim 'we are what we eat'. Southeast Asian spa cuisine adds a bit of oriental pizzazz to healthy dining choices.

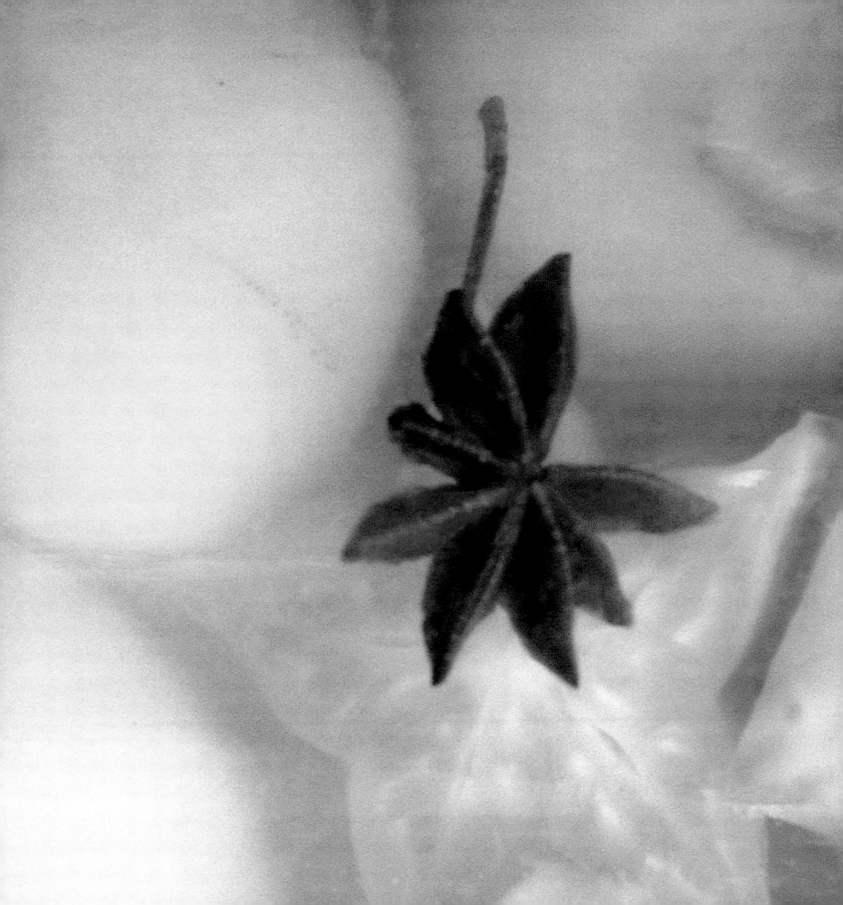

A Kickstart to the Day

As the years roll by, people the world over are getting fatter. This is not because we are eating more. Surveys show that generally people are eating less; they are just eating badly. One of the prime culprits of this is skipping breakfast in the mad dash for the office; culprit number two: a sedentary lifestyle.

When we skip meals we send our bodies into starvation mode forcing them to store up the energy they are not getting and making us feel lethargic as a result. Instead we should eat little and often and prepare our bodies for the rigours of the day with a sensible breakfast that contains unrefined starches, for example the whole grains in muesli. These may take some time for the body to digest, but the nutrients in them are easily absorbed releasing steady levels of energy throughout the day. What's more, people who eat lots of starchy, fibrous foods, including fruit and vegetables, have a lower risk of both heart disease and cancer. Here are some healthy breakfast options, from the *Nusa Dua Spa* in Bali.

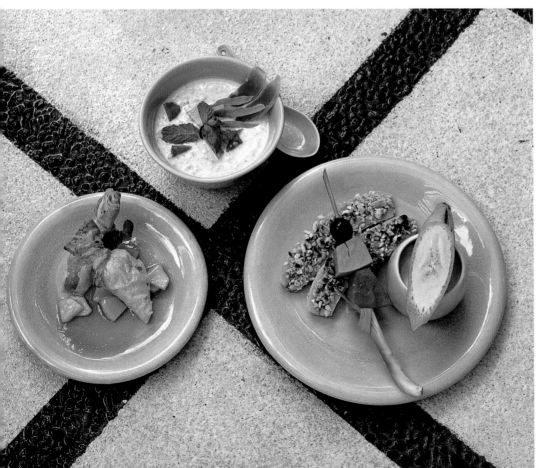

Asian Golden Muesli
(serves four)

250 gms (1 cup)	Swiss muesli
600 ml (3 cups)	soy milk
100 gms (¹/₂ cup)	plain yoghurt
150 gms (³/₄ cup)	papaya, chopped
150 gms (³/₄ cup)	mango, chopped
100 gms (¹/₂ cup)	fructose
juice of 4	limes, juiced
100 gms (¹/₂ cup)	honey
2 ml (1 tsp)	pandan essence (*krim bai toey*, sold at Thai grocery stores)

Method Mix all the ingredients together, then pour into a medium-sized bowl. The mixture can be stored for four hours before serving. If the mixture is a little dry, add more soy milk, then garnish with dry sweet papaya and dry mango and mint leaves.

Grilled Banana with Cashew Nuts and Honey served with Fresh Fruit
(serves four)

4	bananas
80 gms (¹/₄ cup)	honey
88 gms (¹/₄ cup)	cashew nuts, chopped
120 gms (¹/₂ cup)	plain yoghurt
4 gms (2 tsp)	dextrose
40 gms (¹/₄ cup)	tangerine juice
4 sticks	lemon grass
80 gms (¹/₂ cup)	papaya, chopped
60 gms (¹/₂ cup)	watermelon, chopped
20 gms (¹/₄ cup)	grapefruit sections

Method Slice the bananas in half and grill until they are a little soft. Brush with honey and sprinkle with chopped cashew nuts. Grill again until golden brown. Place on a dessert plate with plain yoghurt and the tangerine juice and dextrose mix. Skewer the fresh fruit on to the lemon grass stick, place on the side and serve immediately.

Apple Strudel with Honey
(serves four)

175 gms (2 cups)	apple, chopped
50 gms (6 tbsp)	fructose
2 gms (1 tsp)	cinnamon
40 gms (¹/₄ cup)	raisins
3 gms (2 tsp)	lime juice
2 gms (1 tsp)	zest of lime
25 gms (2 tbsp)	honey
100 gms (1 cup)	breadcrumbs
40 gms (¹/₂ cup)	almonds, ground
25 gms (2 tbsp)	butter
dash	vanilla essence
180 gms (¹/₄ lb)	filo pastry dough
1	egg, lightly whisked

For the Apple Sauce

50 gms (¹/₄ cup)	apple juice
40 gms (¹/₄ cup)	fructose
25 gms (2 tbsp)	honey
5 gms (1 tsp)	flour
50 gms (³/₄ cup)	apple, chopped
60 gms (6 tbsp)	water

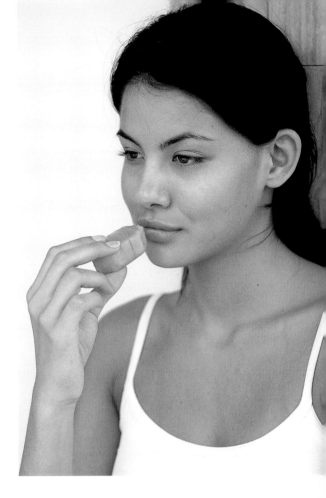

Method Mix all the ingredients, with the exception of the pastry and the egg. Unroll the filo pastry which should be four layers thick. Cut the pastry into four squares. Divide the filling into four parts. Place a ¹/₄ of the filling in the centre of each pastry square. Brush with the egg, then bake for 20 minutes in a preheated oven at 325°F (160°C).

For the sauce, mix all the ingredients together in a food processor. Serve with the apple strudel when fully baked.

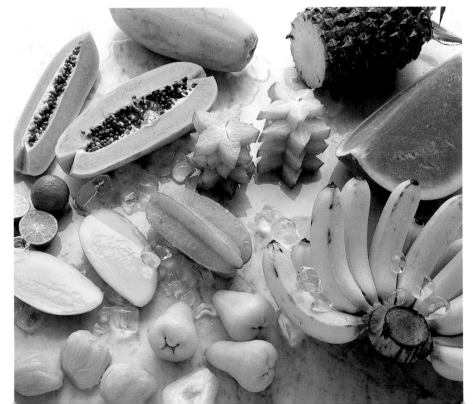

Simple Food

After your body has gone through the rigours of massage it is advisable to eat simple food that is easily digestible. Your digestive system is also much more responsive when you are feeling calm. At *The Serai* in east Bali, the chef creates tasty recipes that require little cooking. These dishes are healthy post-massage snacks that are light without being insubstantial.

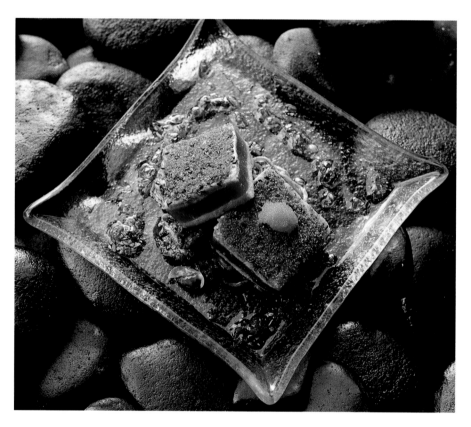

Tuna with Coriander and Ginger Dressing, and Spinach Noodles
(one serving)

1 (6–8 oz)	tuna steak
1 recipe	Pepper Mix (see below)
1 tbsp	vegetable oil
90 gms (¹/₄ lb)	spinach noodles
1 recipe	Coriander and Ginger Dressing (see below)
small bunch	chopped coriander

Pepper Mix Mix together the following: 1 tbsp Cajun spice, 1 tbsp whole black sesame seeds, 1 tbsp (less if dried) fresh oregano, 1 tsp garlic powder, 1 tbsp (less if dried) roasted ground coriander seeds, 1 tsp roasted ground fennel seeds.

Coriander and Ginger Dressing Mix together the following: 4 slices ginger, 450 mls (³/₄ cup) olive oil, 30 mls (1 tbsp) rice wine vinegar, 30 mls (1 tbsp) Mirin (rice wine), 1 clove garlic, salt and pepper to taste.

Method Coat the tuna steak in the Pepper Mix and pan fry in hot vegetable oil for approximately two minutes each side. Blanch the noodles, for about two minutes in boiling water. Drain them well. Serve the tuna on top of the noodles and coat with the Coriander and Ginger Dressing and chopped coriander.

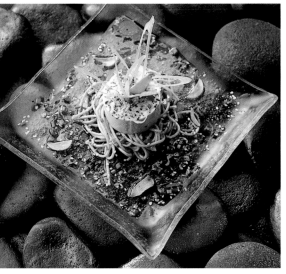

Silken Tofu

(one serving)

75 gms ($^1/_2$ cup)	blanched buckwheat soba noodles
1 recipe	Japanese Ponzu Sauce
half	small red chilli, sliced
1 tsp	sesame oil
1 tsp	lime juice
3 slices	silken tofu (about $^1/_2$ cup)
half	leek, sliced, fried in vegetable oil until crispy
pinch	ground black pepper
small bunch	chopped coriander

Ponzu Sauce Ponzu is a Japanese citrus sauce available in Asian-style grocery stores. Mix one part Ponzu with one part Mirin (rice wine) and one part soy sauce, some crispy fried garlic (do it with the leeks), 1 tbsp olive oil and salt and pepper to taste.

Method Soak the noodles in half of the Ponzu sauce, then add the sesame oil and lime juice and half the chopped coriander. Place the sliced silken tofu on top of the noodles and garnish with the crispy leeks, ground black pepper, rest of the chopped coriander and the remaining Ponzu sauce.

Rucola (Rocket or Arugula) Salad

(one serving)

$^1/_2$ cup	Parmesan cheese, grated
handful	fresh rucola leaves
1 recipe	Balsamic Dressing (see below)

Balsamic Dressing Mix together 150 mls (6 tbsp) olive oil, 50 mls (2 tbsp) balsamic vinegar, $^1/_2$ tsp puréed fresh garlic, salt and pepper to taste.

Method Arrange the grated Parmesan cheese in a rectangle shape roughly 8 cm by 4 cm (4 inches by 2 inches) on grease-proof paper. Bake in a preheated 350°F (170°C) oven until the cheese is golden brown, about 10 minutes. While the cheese is still hot, wrap it around a wine bottle or soft drinks can so it dries in a cylindrical shape; remove when it is cool and firm. Arrange the rucola leaves in the cheese basket; drizzle with the Balsamic Dressing.

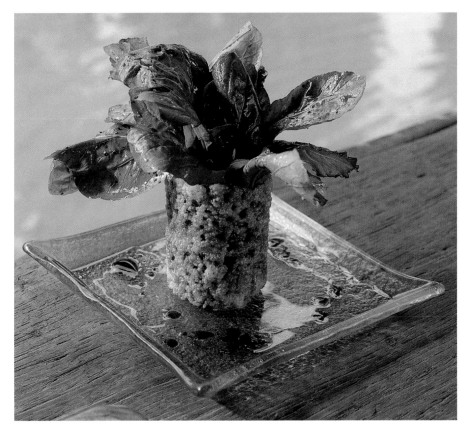

A Natural Feast

One of the many delights of tropical Asia is dining *al fresco*. Food somehow tastes better eaten under a grass roof open at the sides to make the most of a warm evening breeze. At *Begawan Giri Estate* in Ubud, outdoor dining is taken one step further. Order a designer picnic and find a secluded spot amongst some of Bali's most dramatic, landscaped scenery.

Here, a poolside snack is given new meaning. Chips and pizza wedges round the lap pool are swapped for a bit of banana blossom and a bamboo salad at the edge of a jungle rock pool, fed via a waterfall from a 'holy' spring. You feel like a wood nymph as you nibble away in nirvana!

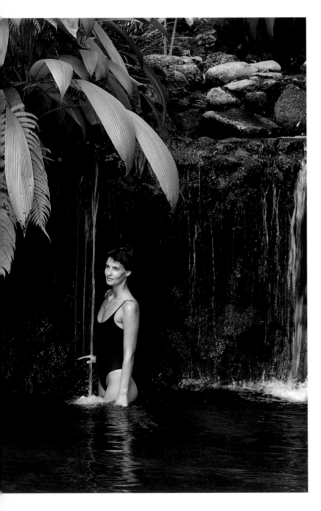

Asparagus and Oyster Mushroom Salad
(one serving)

4 spears	asparagus
6	oyster mushrooms
60 gms (4 tbsp)	fresh coconut, shredded
60 gms (4 tbsp)	lemon grass, finely sliced
15 gms (1 tbsp)	lime leaves, finely sliced
15 gms (1 tbsp)	red shallots, finely sliced
60 gms (4 tbsp)	mint leaves
60 gms (4 tbsp)	coriander leaves
1 recipe	Dressing (see below)
2 gms (¹/₂ tbsp)	sesame seeds
2	starfruit leaves (or basil leaves), crisply fried

Dressing

60 gms (4 tbsp)	coconut cream
30 gms (2 tbsp)	Chilli Jam (see right)
15 gms (1 tbsp)	palm sugar
30 gms (2 tbsp)	fish sauce (*nam pla*)
2 small	green chillies, sliced
2 tbsp	Kaffir lime or kalamansi lime juice

To make the Dressing Lightly whisk all ingredients together.

To make Chilli Jam Fry, in 60 ml (4 tbsp) grapeseed oil, 60 gms (4 tbsp) sliced red shallots, and strain; then 30 gms (2 tbsp) sliced garlic; then 15 gms (1 tbsp) dried shrimps; 15 gms (1 tbsp) de-seeded dried chilli (for only 10 seconds). Slice 5 gms (1 tbsp) galangal (or ginger, as a substitute) and pan-toast until perfumed and slightly charred. Cool these ingredients, then blend or purée together with the strained oil. Return the paste to a pot and cook until aromatic and a deep shiny black colour.

Finally, season with 20 gms (1¹/₂ tbsp) fish sauce (*nam pla*), 15 ml (1 tbsp) palm sugar and 15 ml (1 tbsp) tamarind water (this is obtained by covering tamarind pulp with warm/hot water, allowing it to seep for 30 minutes, then literally pushing the solids through a strainer). A jam consistency will now have been achieved.

Method Blanch asparagus in chicken stock or water and slice into three pieces. Char-grill the oyster mushroom. To assemble, tumble all the ingredients together, add the Dressing and sprinkle with sesame seeds and crisply fried starfruit leaves.

Crisp Banana Blossom and Green Apple Salad

(one serving)

60 gms (4 tbsp)	banana blossom
60 gms (4 tbsp)	green apple, julienned
15 gms (1 tbsp)	red shallot, sliced
15 gms (1 tbsp)	red shallot, char-grilled
15 gms (1 tbsp)	mint leaves
15 gms (1 tbsp)	coriander leaves
15 gms (1 tbsp)	sliced garlic, crisp-fried
15 gms (1 tbsp)	sliced shallot, crisp-fried
1 recipe	Batter (see below)
1 recipe	Dressing (see below)

Batter Mix together 12 gms (8 tbsp) rice flour, 60 gms (4 tbsp) corn flour, 120 ml (8 tbsp) water and a pinch of salt.

Dressing

1	large red chilli
60 gms (4 tbsp)	lime juice
60 gms (4 tbsp)	orange juice
15 gms (1 tbsp)	white sugar
15 ml (1 tbsp)	fish sauce (*nam pla*)

To make the Dressing Pound in a mortar and pestle the large red chilli until fine. Add all remaining ingredients, stand for 10 mins, stirring lightly on occasion.

Method Top off the round end of the banana flower and peel down the red outer leaves until the white heart appears. Slice it lengthways into four and remove from each piece the hard inner stem. Shake out the flower spores between each layer. Slice the blossom very finely lengthways, working quickly to avoid discolouration. Immediately place in the batter and fry in hot oil over a high heat. Lift out and drain. Finish the salad, by folding all ingredients together.

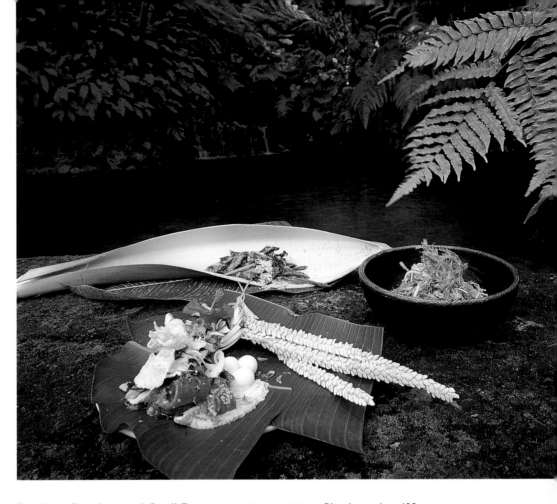

Bamboo, Eggplant and Quail Eggs with a Peanut Relish

(one serving)

1	capsicum
1	baby eggplant
3	quail eggs
30 gms (2 tbsp)	fresh bamboo, cooked in water for 30-40 mins
20 gms (1 1/2 tbsp)	silken tofu, uncooked
1 tsp	fried crisp shallots
60 gms (4 tbsp)	snake beans, blanched in salted water
4	melinjo nut wafers
1 recipe	Peanut Relish

Peanut Relish Blend together 400 gms (2 cups) char-grilled red shallots, 400 gms (2 cups) char-grilled garlic, 60 gms (1/4 cup) finely chopped galangal, 120 gms (1/2 cup) finely chopped lemon grass, 1 large dried chilli soaked in hot water for 30 mins, and then fry with a little vegetable oil for 40 minutes on a low heat. Add 1 cup peanuts, boiled for 10 mins and strained, 1 tsp lime juice and 1 tsp dark palm sugar.

Method Peel and de-seed the capsicum and char-grill. Slice and deep-fry the eggplant. Soft boil the eggs for 2 1/2 minutes. Place the peanut relish on the plate then layer with the above ingredients, followed by the bamboo, tofu, shallots and beans, adding the melinjo wafers at the end.

Tasteful Thai

Guests at *Chiva-Som* have no choice but to reassess their eating habits. Everyone here is presented with a low-fat, no-salt menu three times a day. While Thai food has historically been healthy, it has developed over the years to rely heavily on fat-filled coconut milk, coconut oil and pork meat. *Chiva-Som*'s healthy alternatives are high on flavour and low on these villains. Salt is substituted with soy or fish sauce (*nam pla*) and frying is done with vegetable stock rather than with oil. When using vegetable stock continue adding two tablespoons throughout the cooking process, maintaining the same high heat as if using oil. Here's how:

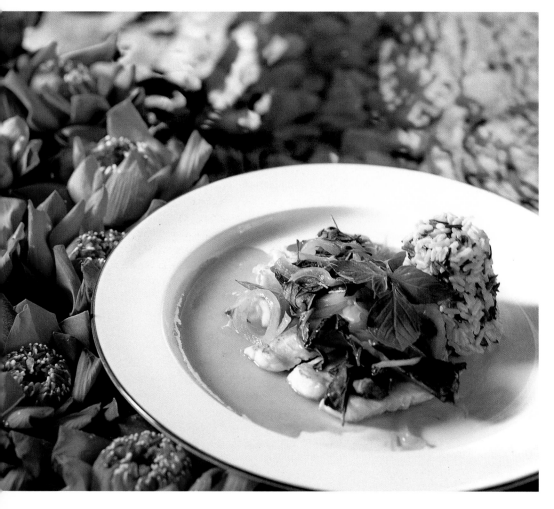

Stir Fried King Fish Thai Style

(serves four)

600 gms (1 1/2 lb)	king fish fillet (or other white fish)
2 cloves	garlic
1	small onion
2	green chilli or red chilli
2 tsp	fresh Thai basil
150 mls (1/2 cup)	vegetable stock
2 tbsp	fish sauce (*nam pla*) or light soy sauce
200 gms (1 cup)	brown rice

Method Steam the brown rice until crispy, but not overcooked. Cut the fish into medallions, about 1 cm x 3 cm. Crush the garlic and peel and shred the onion. Finely slice the green chilli (or shred the red chilli depending on what you use). Heat a wok or heavy frying pan until hot (but not smoking). Add 50 ml of the stock, the shredded onion and crushed garlic and cook quickly, stirring continuously to prevent burning. If this becomes too dry add a little more stock. Add the fish and continue to stir for 3–4 minutes, taking care not to break up the fish. Continue to add a little stock if the mixture becomes too dry. Add the chilli and basil with the fish sauce. Mix well to coat the fish and serve with the brown rice.

Thai Seafood Salad

(serves four)

4 cloves	garlic
12	bird's-eye chillis
8 tbsp (¹/₄ cup)	lemon juice
4 tsp	fish sauce (*nam pla*)
1 tsp	honey
4 thin strips	lemon grass
400 gms (1 lb)	mixed, cooked seafood
4	tomatoes
2 stalks	celery
1	large onion
4	spring onions
40 gms (2 tbsp)	Chinese parsley (cilantro)

Method Crush the garlic and chilli together. Add the fish sauce, lemon juice, sliced lemon grass and honey. Set aside. Mix the cooked seafood with the finely shredded celery and onion, seeded and sliced tomato, spring onions and parsley, then mix together with the dressing. Serve immediately.

Lentil Wontons with Sweet and Sour Sauce, Thai Style

(serves four)

75 gms (1 cup)	dry lentils
2 tsp	soy sauce
3	spring onions, chopped
¹/₂ tsp	fresh, grated ginger
32	wonton wrappers
1 recipe	Sweet and Sour Sauce
750 ml (2¹/₂ cups)	vegetable stock

Sweet and Sour Sauce

125 mls (¹/₂ cup)	vegetable stock
¹/₄	pineapple, diced
¹/₄	cucumber, seeded and diced
¹/₂	bell pepper, chopped
2	tomatoes, seeded
1	spring onion, chopped
2	small chilli
2 tsp	soy sauce
¹/₂ tsp	corn starch
to taste	salt and pepper

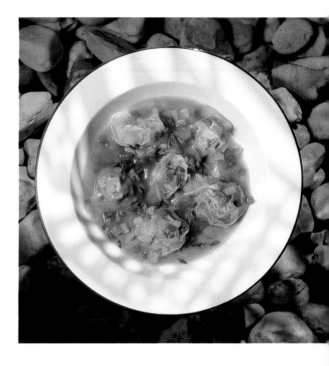

Method Cook the lentils, then mash the cooked lentils in a bowl and add the soy, spring onions and ginger. Place a teaspoonful in the centre of each wonton wrapper and fold up, moistening the edges with water to seal and shape. Blanch these for 2–3 minutes. Meanwhile, mix the sauce ingredients. Boil the wontons in the vegetable stock, cooking thoroughly for 2–3 minutes. Drain and place in the centre of a plate. Pour over the sauce to serve.

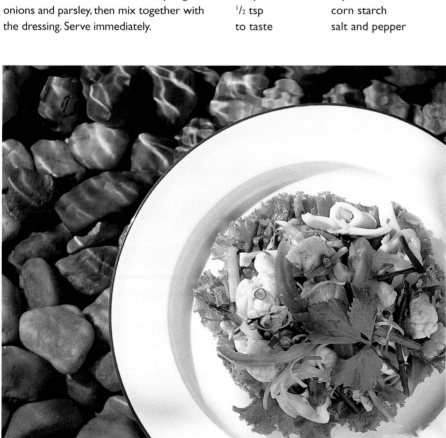

Dining Light

Not many of us manage to stick by the rules of healthy eating, especially when it comes to dinner which, nutritionists tell us, should be eaten at least three hours before bedtime. However we can avoid system overload in our slumbering hours by eating sensibly after dark. This means eating foods that are easily digestible, foods that are as near to their natural state as possible and foods that, if not raw, are lightly cooked: preferably steamed or grilled so that their nutrients are not zapped or strangled by heavy sauces. We should put a hold on our portion size, eat slowly and masticate!

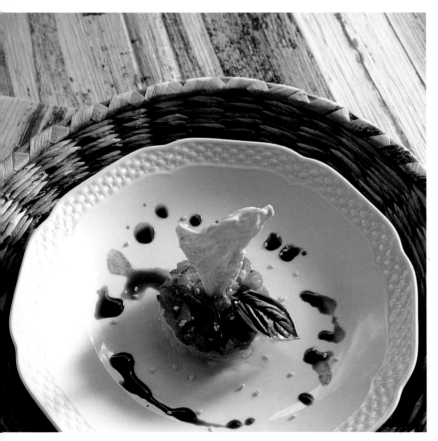

Don't worry about clock watching if you take this evening meal on the lip of Ayung River Gorge at The Chedi in Ubud, Bali, where the location alone will set you up to eat properly – and slowly – and sleep blissfully afterwards.

Tuna Tartar With Cucumber Yoghurt Sauce
(one serving)

75 gms (3 oz)	fresh red tuna (sashimi grade)
20 gms (1 tbsp)	pickled ginger slices
1 tsp	fresh ginger juice, squeezed from grated ginger
3–4 ($^1/_4$ cup)	spring onions, chopped into small rings
$^1/_8$ tsp	Wasabi paste
1 tbsp	soy sauce
1 recipe	Cucumber Yoghurt Sauce (see below)
to garnish	shredded cucumber, sesame seed cracker, sesame seeds

Cucumber Yoghurt Sauce Mix together 1 tbsp yoghurt, 2 tbsp puréed cucumber (seeds removed), salt and pepper to taste.

Method Cut the tuna into small cubes. Mix the Wasabi paste and soy sauce until smooth. Toss the tuna with the Wasabi and soy and the other ingredients until well mixed. On a plate pack the shredded cucumber garnish half way up a metal or pastry ring. Tightly stack the tuna mixture on top to form a cylindrical structure. Pour a circle of cucumber yoghurt sauce around the tuna. Remove the ring. Sprinkle with sesame seeds and serve with a sesame seed cracker on top.

Grilled Chicken Teriyaki and Spicy Noodle Salad

(one serving)

150 gms (5 oz)	chicken breast, boneless and skinless
125 gms ($^1/_2$ cup)	soba noodles
30 gms (2 tbsp)	carrots, shredded
25 gms ($^1/_4$ cup)	broccoli florets
15 gms ($^1/_2$)	leek, julienned
20 gms (2 tbsp)	snowpea pods
15 gms (1 tbsp)	pickled ginger, julienned
$^1/_8$ tsp	Wasabi paste
5 gms (2 tbsp)	nori, shredded in strips
1 recipe	Teriyaki Sauce (see below)
1 recipe	Dressing (see below)

Teriyaki Sauce Mix together 7 tsp soy sauce, 2 tsp sugar, 1 tsp chopped garlic, 1 tsp chopped ginger, 7 tsp Saké and 7 tsp Mirin.

Dressing Mix together 1 tbsp rice vinegar, 1 tbsp Kikkoman soy sauce, 2 tbsp Mirin, 1 tbsp sesame oil, 1 tsp Saké and 2 tbsp chilli oil.

Method Marinate the chicken breast in the Teriyaki Sauce for at least two hours. Cook the noodles until al dente, approximately two minutes. Cool them down in iced water and drain them. Keep aside. Blanch all the vegetables. Grill the chicken breast and slice. Toss the noodles with the vegetables, pickled ginger and Wasabi. Pile them all into a spiral. Top with the chicken pieces and nori strips and sprinkle Dressing and sesame seeds on top.

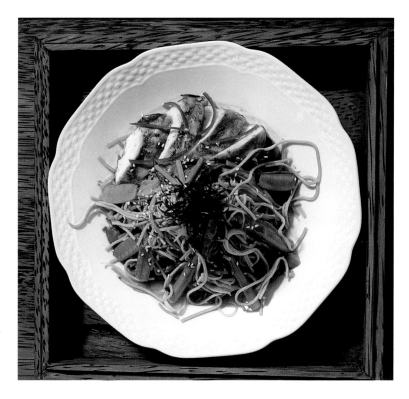

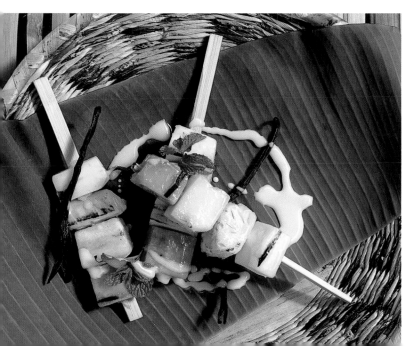

Grilled Fruit Skewers with Honey Yoghurt Sauce

(one serving)

2–3 slices	pineapple, peeled and cored
1	banana
$^1/_2$	papaya
$^1/_4$	melon, seeded
1 tsp	honey
1 tsp	lime juice
1 tbsp	butter
1 recipe	Honey Yoghurt Sauce (see below)
to garnish	mint

Honey Yoghurt Sauce Mix together 2 tsps yoghurt, 1 tsp honey, seeds scraped from 1 vanilla bean, 1 gm ($^1/_4$ tsp) ground cinnamon.

Method Cut the fruit into large cubes of equal size and skewer them. Brush them with lime juice and a bit of honey (optional). Then brush with butter and grill. Try to get sear marks from the hot grill. Drizzle the sauce over the skewers and garnish with sprigs of mint.

Liquid Assets

Everybody knows that healthy eating is a metaphor for feeling great and living longer but the adage "you are what you drink" hasn't caught on with the same fervour. The daily prescription for two litres of water somehow never makes the leap from our minds to our gullets. But it is in fact drinking good quality fluids regularly that has the most important impact on our general health. And it doesn't just have to be water – spring, filtered or distilled. Here are some other options:

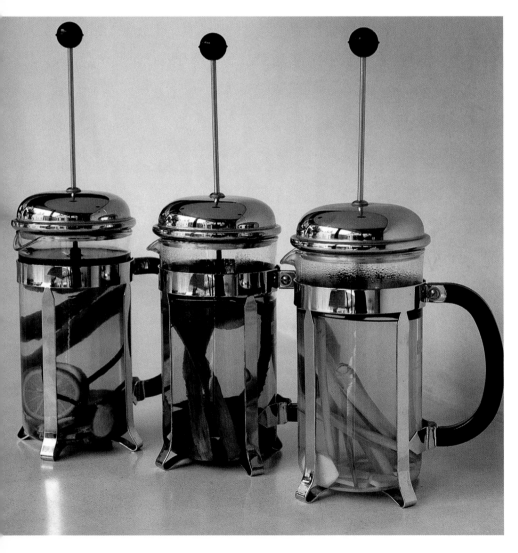

Herbal teas and freshly squeezed juices inject us with just as much vitality as health-giving foods. Such fluids flush out unwanted toxins and help re-hydrate the body's organs, increasing blood flow and moving oxygen more efficiently around the body. In this respect they are ideal for topping off the benefits of a body treatment or massage.

Natural juices and smoothies, containing yoghurt or milk with puréed fresh fruit, have become part of the healthy eating lexicon because they are excellent meal substitutes and that much more easy to digest than solid foods. They are perfect spa food because they satisfy our mild hunger pangs after treatments without overloading the system. Fruit, in particular, is easily digestible and cleansing while containing fructose, which gives energy. It also has a cooling, calming action on the body and has that all-important high water content.

Both fruit and vegetables are important sources of anti-oxidant vitamins and minerals which zap free radicals, those harmful molecules that damage cells and cause premature ageing and such conditions as cancer, heart disease, arthritis and diabetes. The most important vitamins found naturally in fruits are vitamins A, C and E. But besides all its health giving properties, fruit, whizzed into a thick, tangy pulp, with or without milk and yoghurt, is so deliciously refreshing that it's usually gone in a gulp.

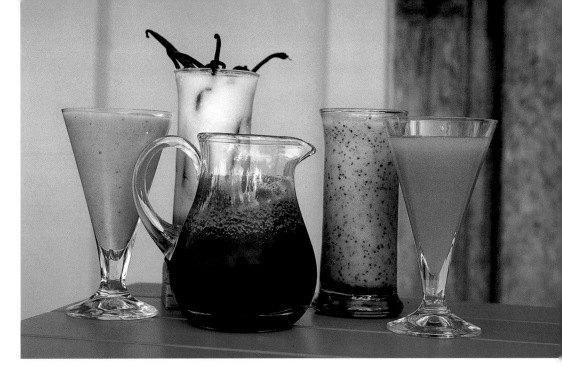

Herbal Infusions

Herbal teas started with the Greeks and Romans and were drunk all over the world until the 1940s when Western medicine became overrun with science and frowned upon any alternative approach. By contrast, infusions of herbs and spices have always had a role in oriental diet for the mild effect they can have on stimulating the kidneys, calming digestion, aiding circulation and, of course, putting water back into our bodies (this we apparently lose at a rate of 1.8 litres per day).

Discard the dusty tea bags that start off bland and become stale in favour of loose-leaf herbs and spices in their natural state. You can concoct a variety of teas to suit your mood and your taste buds. Try some camomile for stress, nettle for skin problems, garlic or peppermint for bronchitis, ginger for tummy trouble and raspberry leaf in preparation for labour.

Some popular infusions from *The Serai* in east Bali are pictured left:

Ginger and lemon grass – a stomach settler and tonic for pregnant women; it also helps with motion sickness.
Cinnamon, ginger and lime leaf – for warming the body in cool weather, with mild astringent properties.
Vanilla, cinnamon, lime fruit, turmeric and ginger – ginger and turmeric are blood cleansers and stomach settlers; the vanilla adds flavour and the lime has acidic and cleansing properties.

Thirst-Quenchers
From *The Spa at Jimbaran*, Four Seasons Resort, Bali

Tropical Passion – passion fruit, orange, banana and lime juice
Coconilla – cool coconut water and milk with vanilla beans
Blushing Beat – beetroot, cucumber and fresh lime
Guava Gulp – mango, guava nectar, banana and lime juice
Jamu Wanita – Javanese herbal drink believed to clean the blood, improve vitality and act as an aphrodisiac!

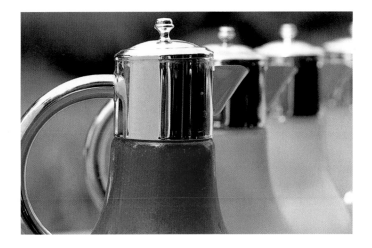

Just Juices
From *The Datai*, Langkawi
Watermelon juice, Orange juice, Guava juice and Melon juice.

Herbal Tonics

Jamu is one of the greatest success stories of the beauty industry, yet it is virtually unknown outside its country of origin, Indonesia. In that country, 80 percent of the population relies on its natural medicinal powers to attain the figure, the complexion, the physical strength or the mood they desire. Broadly speaking, jamu refers to any kind of traditional medicine. But most people think of jamu as a herbal beverage with medicinal qualities and swig back a daily glass to achieve their heart's desire – or a few more glasses to cure an ailment already there.

The origins of jamu are lost in time, though, like most of the country's beauty rituals, it is supposed to have been born in the in central Java where commercial production is still based. The purest forms of jamu come from the island of Madura, where women reputedly can live to 135 years of age.

In fairytale fashion the magic jamu potions – herbs, roots, barks, leaves, honey, fruits, egg yolk and 'other ingredients' – are handed down verbally from mother to daughter through the generations. It is very much a woman's industry.

While the more common mixtures are taken for general health, strength and beauty, there are more than 350 well-known recipes for conditions as varied as skin whitening, kidney stones, malaria and flu. Most popular jamus contain turmeric for its astringent qualities and tamarind for flavour and blood cleansing. The dried ingredients are usually mixed with water plus a little honey or lime to taste. Under commercial production, the potent plant matter is ground into powder and pill form for convenience. However, a bag of dried herbs from Madura still has the greatest effect and stays potent for five years.

Visit *Hotel Tugu* in Bali for access to the best jamu available (see recipes below and right). Not only does this spa have a hot line to Madura, they make the traditional tonics on site. Most of Indonesia's spas offer more palatable jamus for general wellbeing. Drink one before or during your treatment to warm and prepare your body.

Jamu Koeat Lelaki (Strong Man Jamu)

This is a man's jamu. It makes one glass. It is taken to enhance vitality and endurance in bed. For continual high performance, a glass should be drunk morning and evening.

1 tbsp	black pepper, crushed
1 tbsp	coffee beans, ground
100 gms (2 tbsp)	ginger juice, from soaked, shredded ginger
3 tbsp	honey
juice of 1	lime, juiced
1	free-range egg

Method Put all the ingredients into a glass and mix. Cover with half a glass of hot water and drink down immediately.

Jamu Koenci Seoroeh

This is a women's jamu: it eliminates body odour, reduces the intensity of both period and period pains and is taken to keep the body tight and youthful. It can be drunk, like water, any time. The following recipe makes five bottles of jamu, or three days supply.

200 gms (1 cup)	Chinese keys (*Boesenbergia pandurata*)
100 gms (6 tbsp)	galangal (or ginger)
100 gms (6 tbsp)	turmeric, ground
3 tbsp	coriander, ground
handful	betel leaves (*Piper betle*)
200 gms (1 cup)	pressed tamarind
500 gms (1 lb)	coconut sugar
150 gms (6 tbsp)	white sugar
3 litres (3 quarts)	drinking water
to taste	salt

Method Clean, peel and cut the Chinese keys, galangal and turmeric. Put these together in a juicer with the coriander and betel leaves and water. After blending, strain. Soak the tamarind in warm water and strain it to get the juice. Mix the coconut sugar and white sugar together in boiled water and strain. Combine all the above in a bowl and add salt to taste before serving. The amount produced can be kept for up to one week in the fridge.

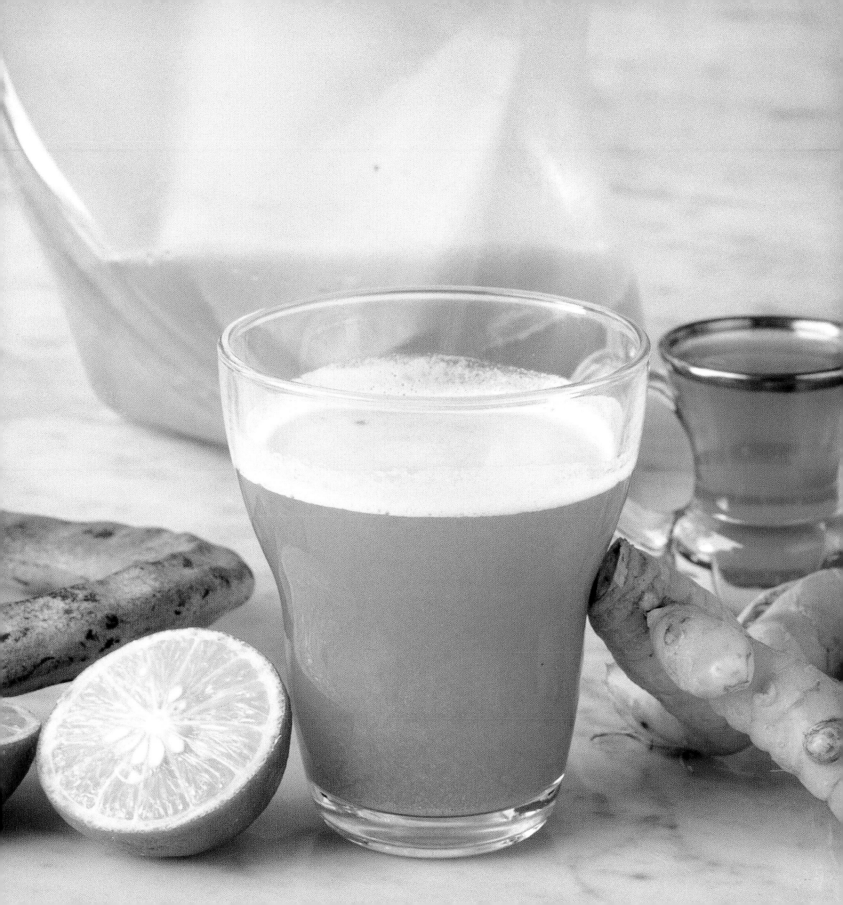

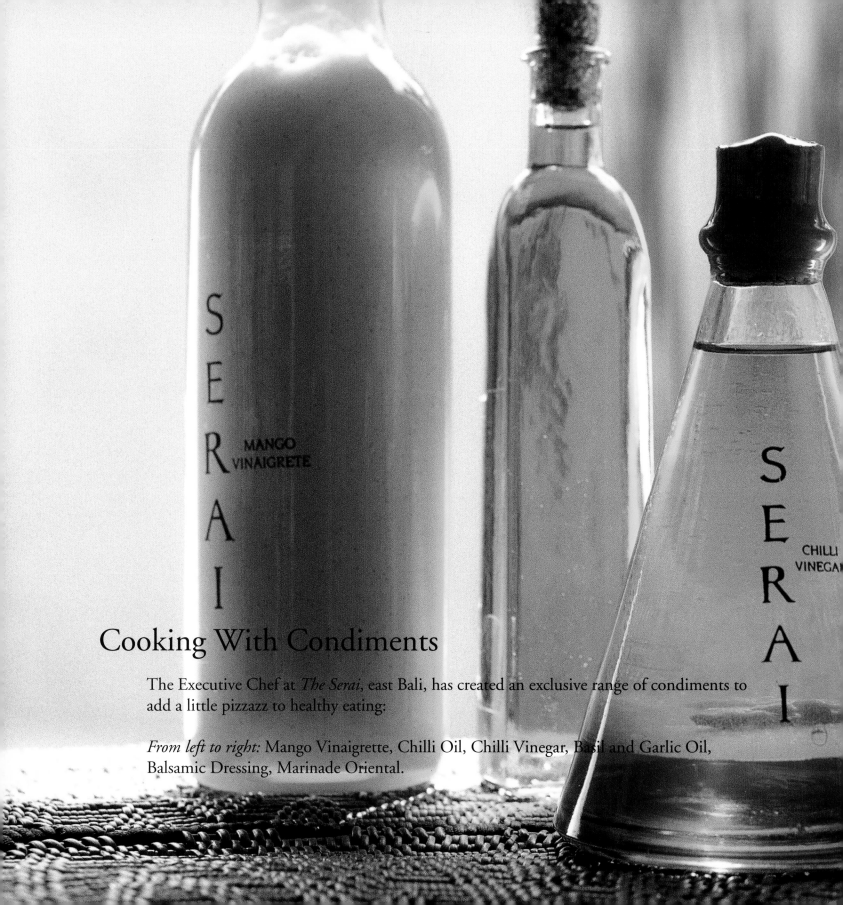

Cooking With Condiments

The Executive Chef at *The Serai*, east Bali, has created an exclusive range of condiments to add a little pizzazz to healthy eating:

From left to right: Mango Vinaigrette, Chilli Oil, Chilli Vinegar, Basil and Garlic Oil, Balsamic Dressing, Marinade Oriental.

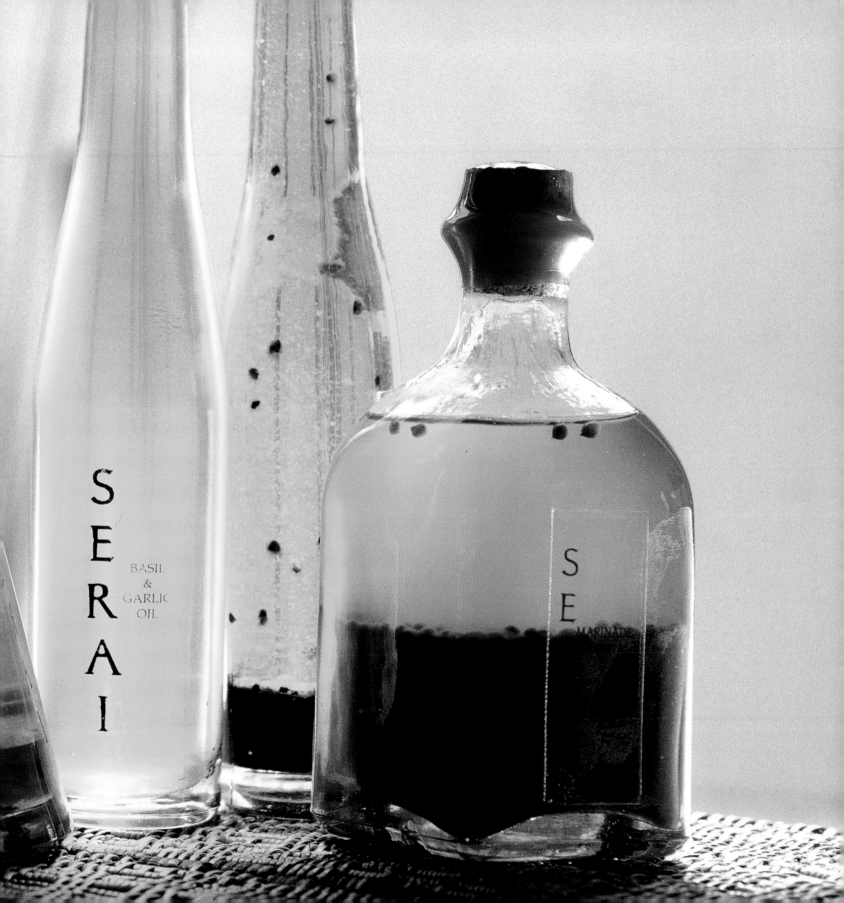

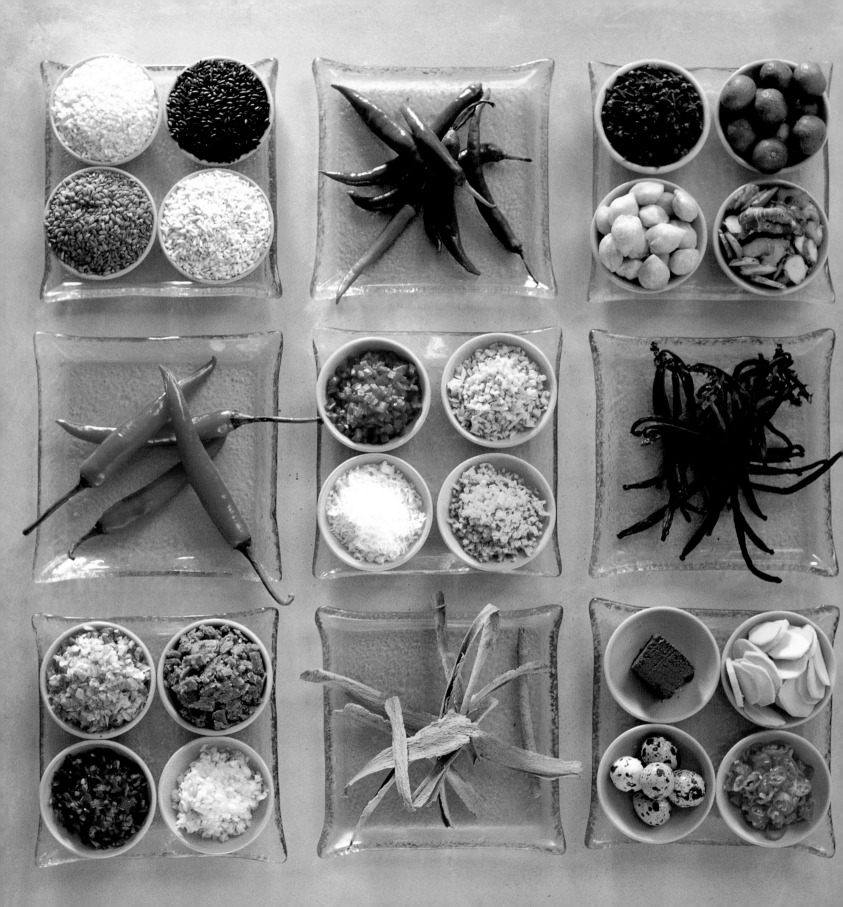

natural spa ingredients

The enormous wealth of natural eco-systems makes southeast Asia a botanical treasure trove. The medicinal qualities of much of its abundant plant life have, for centuries, formed the backbone of health and beauty therapy throughout this huge and exotic continent. Such is the potency of nature in this part of the world that it has found favour in beauty salons everywhere. Here we list some of the most common natural ingredients used.

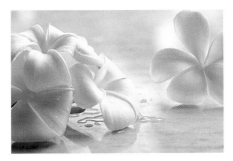

FRANGIPANI or **PLUMERIA** (*Plumeria sp.*) is one of the most prolific flowers in tropical Asia. The waxy, aromatic blooms fall constantly from the tree of the same name; consequently, they are commonly used in offerings and ceremonies and to decorate religious icons. The plumeria tree is often planted on grave sites in the region.

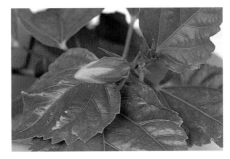

The **HIBISCUS LEAF** (*Hibiscus sp.*) is the sole ingredient of a traditional form of shampoo. When they are crushed and boiled in a little water, the leaves' sap forms a sticky, dark-coloured paste that has cleansing properties. The leaf has also traditionally been used as a cleanser in a variety of skin care preparations.

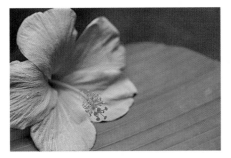

HIBISCUS FLOWERS (*Hibiscus sp.*) are believed to hold certain supernatural powers which absorb negativity and bad spells. The traditional red, orange, yellow and pink blooms have a sweet nectar. They are used for ornamentation purposes and are often found on religious statues. They are also used as an emollient in skin care.

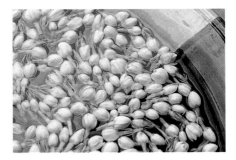

JASMINE (*Jasminum sp.*) is another of tropical Asia's most sweet-smelling flowers. In Thailand, it is a symbol of friendship, and is often strung into garlands and offered to people as a welcome gift and to Buddha as a sign of gratitude. This tiny bud is woven into hair for wedding ceremonies in Java.

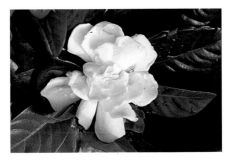

TROPICAL GARDENIA (*Gardenia jasminoides*) is regarded almost as an emblem of the tropics, due to its beautifully strong aroma. In many tropical Asian households, the blooms are put in a bowl of water and displayed in the home where their strong scent permeates into the environment.

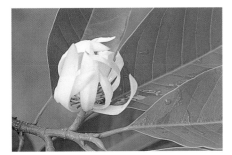

TROPICAL MAGNOLIA or **CHAMPAK** (*Michelia champaca*) is renowned for its cooling and healing powers with specific anti-malarial properties. Its petite web of elegant white petals exudes a scent as sweet as syrup. Like most of her sisters, it is used in prayer ritual and for bathing.

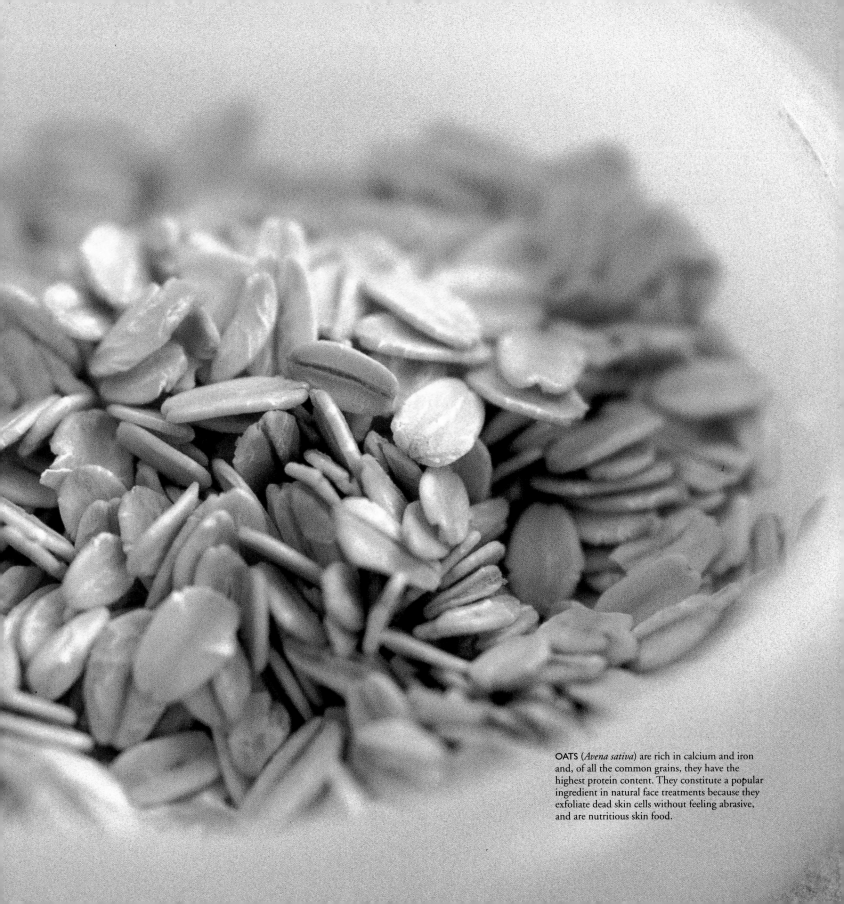

OATS (*Avena sativa*) are rich in calcium and iron and, of all the common grains, they have the highest protein content. They constitute a popular ingredient in natural face treatments because they exfoliate dead skin cells without feeling abrasive, and are nutritious skin food.

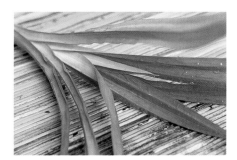

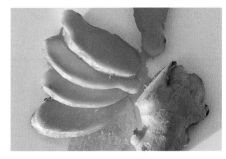

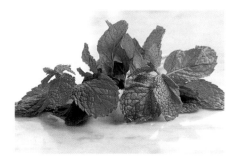

PANDANUS LEAF (*Pandanus amaryllifolius*) is a versatile leaf grown in most gardens, *apotik hidup* (which translates as the 'healing pharmacy') in Indonesia. Thanks to its earthy and sweet aroma this practical leaf is a popular base for cakes and is infused into oils for hair and skin care. It is also used in virtually all Balinese offerings to the Gods.

GINGER (*Zingiber officinale*) is eaten cooked or infused raw into drinks, as a remedy for stomach aches and menstrual pains. Myth says that ginger is key to assisting man's endurance in love-making due to the phallic shape of the rhizome! Used externally, ginger is applied to the body to relieve aching muscles and increase blood circulation.

MINT (*Mentha arvensis*) is a blood cleansing plant because it is antiseptic and antibacterial. It is most commonly taken as a tea simply by infusing a few leaves in boiling water, in order to help clear the complexion. It is also mixed with the crème bath conditioner and rubbed into the scalp to combat dandruff and stimulate hair follicles for growth.

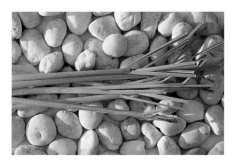

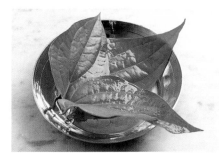

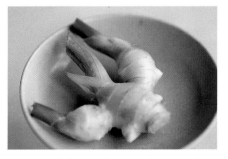

LEMON GRASS (*Cymbopogon citratus*) is a key flavouring in Asian cuisine, resembling lemon rind more closely than the juice. The swollen base of the stem is used, but the whole stalk should be soaked before use. It is eaten to speed up a slow digestive system; its oil is good for calming hot, perspiring feet. Burn the oil for an effective room deodorizer.

BETEL LEAF (*Piper betle*) is an astringent leaf, associated with feminine cleanliness: it is used as a sanitary wipe and as a cleanser when added to bath water. The fresh leaves are cooling on a hot body. It makes a bitter tea believed to help 'dry the vagina' and purify the blood. Both the nut and the leaf are also chewed for a mild stimulating effect.

GALANGAL (*Alpinia galanga*) is a rhizome in the ginger family. It has a complex and earthy taste and a pungency and tang quite unlike common ginger. It is most commonly used in cooking, but its faint aroma of camphor makes it one of the spices used in traditional, warming body scrubs such as the Indonesian *boreh*.

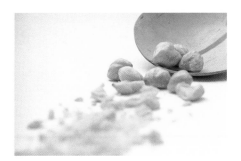

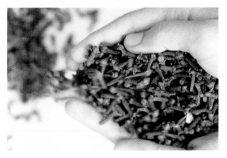

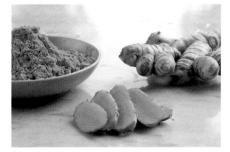

CANDLENUT (*Aleurites moluccana*) is used in cooking across the Asian region. In skincare, the nut's soft and oily consistency makes it a wonderful 'scrub' ingredient. It also acts as soap because, when rubbed over the skin, it draws out impurities and, as proof, changes from creamy to dirty in colour.

CLOVES (*Eugenia caryophyllus*) have analgesic qualities and are traditionally used for pain relief, especially for toothache. They are also antiseptic, increase overall blood circulation and, when chewed, can stop excessive flatulence! Suck a clove when you are tired or stressed or want to give up smoking.

TURMERIC (*Curcuma domestica*) is a basic item in folk medicine in tropical Asia. It is used internally and externally for its astringent and cleansing properties and is a core ingredient for jamu herbal tonics in Indonesia. Its vivid colour gives the Javanese *lulur* (body scrub) its signature orange hue.

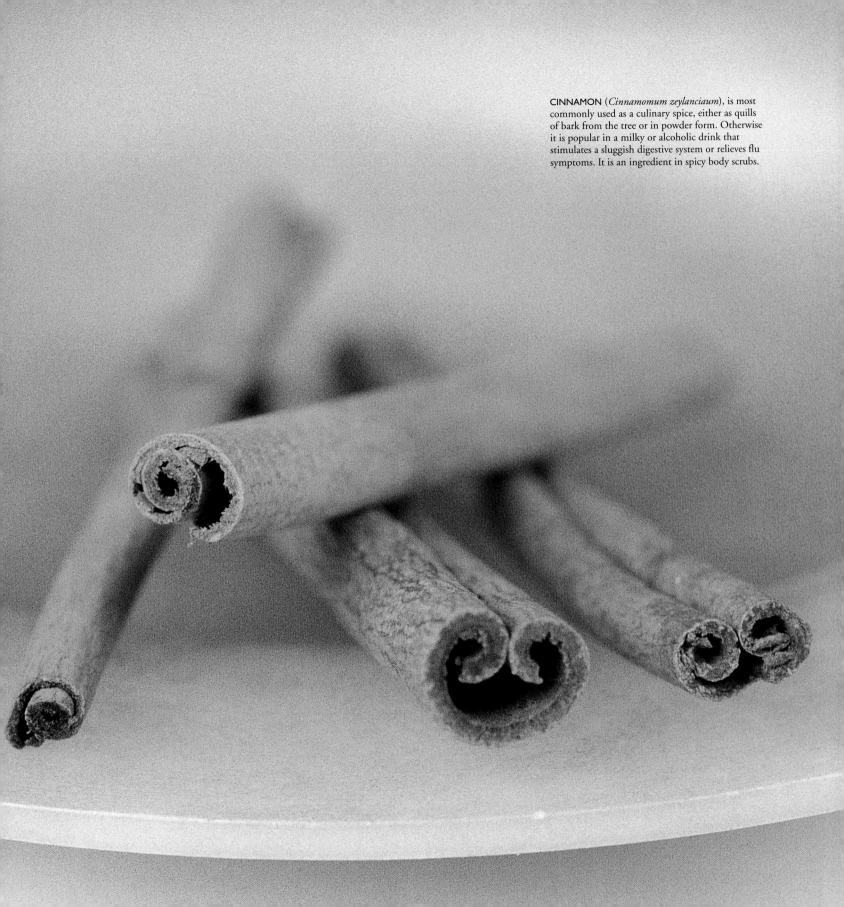

CINNAMON (*Cinnamomum zeylanciaum*), is most commonly used as a culinary spice, either as quills of bark from the tree or in powder form. Otherwise it is popular in a milky or alcoholic drink that stimulates a sluggish digestive system or relieves flu symptoms. It is an ingredient in spicy body scrubs.

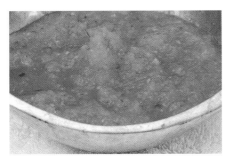

CUCUMBER (*Cucumis sativus*) is used extensively in beauty products as a cooling and revitalizing agent, and is especially effective for oily skin types: its juice makes a good skin tonic and tightens the pores. Cucumber slices on the eyes refresh and moisturize and, for those who forgot their SPF, mashed cucumber soothes sunburnt skin.

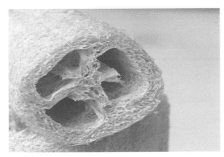

NATURAL SPONGE, otherwise known as 'loofah', is the dried body of the green *gambas* plant. Its fibrous yet gentle constituency makes it ideal for removing dead skin cells while still softening and refreshing the skin. The loofah body scrub, often combined with sea salt and oil, is popular at Thai spas for those who want to invigorate their skin.

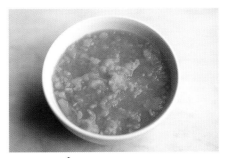

PAPAYA (*Carica papaya*), abundant throughout tropical Asia, contains vitamins (particularly high in A and C) that heal upset stomachs. It contains enzymes which give it mild exfoliating properties, so Asian women daub papaya around their eyes to eradicate fine lines. Alternatively, papaya skins can be rubbed over the face to remove dead skin cells.

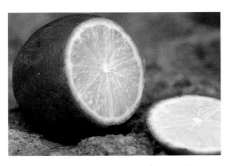

LIME (*Citrus sp*) is used in drinks, food, medicines and beauty regimes throughout southeast Asia. It is high in vitamin C and its astringent qualities make it an effective blood purifier. It is mixed with crushed sea shells and smeared over the stomach as part of traditional slimming ritual and is said to be effective in shrinking the uterus after childbirth.

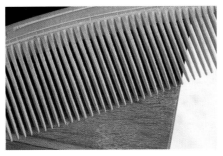

SANDALWOOD (*Santalum sp*) is the most sacred and fragrant of woods, preserved for burning in temple ceremonies. Its heavy, sweet and woody aroma is instantly recognized. In beauty, it is the hallmark of oriental perfume, although it is also believed to calm skin irritations, such as eczema and abscesses, thanks to its astringent properties.

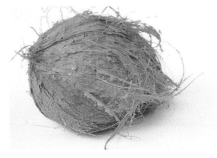

COCONUT (*Cocos nucifera*) is used in countless ways: for eating, drinking, as an ingredient in cakes and as tropical Asia's most prevalent cooking oil. Oil from mature fruit is massaged into the head for soft and shiny hair while the thick white milk is traditionally used as a shampoo and the young, thin milk as a conditioning rinse.

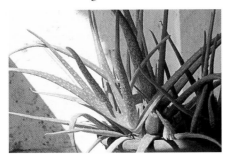

ALOE VERA (*Aloe vera* syn. *Aloe barbadensis*) is much prized for the miraculous healing qualities of the thick, clear liquid stored in its leaves. It is used externally to clear skin blemishes, scars and heal burns or sunburn; internally it may be taken in tablet form for digestive complaints.

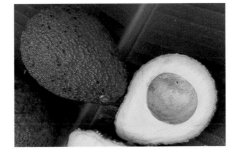

AVOCADO (*Persea americana*) is popular in natural beauty practice because the rich consistency of its flesh and oil, high in vitamin E, is a nourishing skin food, especially effective for dry complexions and brittle hair. Avocados were introduced to southeast Asia two centuries ago from America.

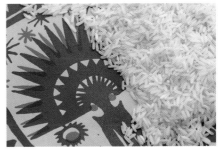

RICE is not just a food, it is a culture and a way of life. Paddies dominate the Indonesian landscape where 8,000 varieties are believed to be grown. Rice is food for half the world's population and, in beauty ritual, is used as a base in body scrubs due to its exfoliating properties.

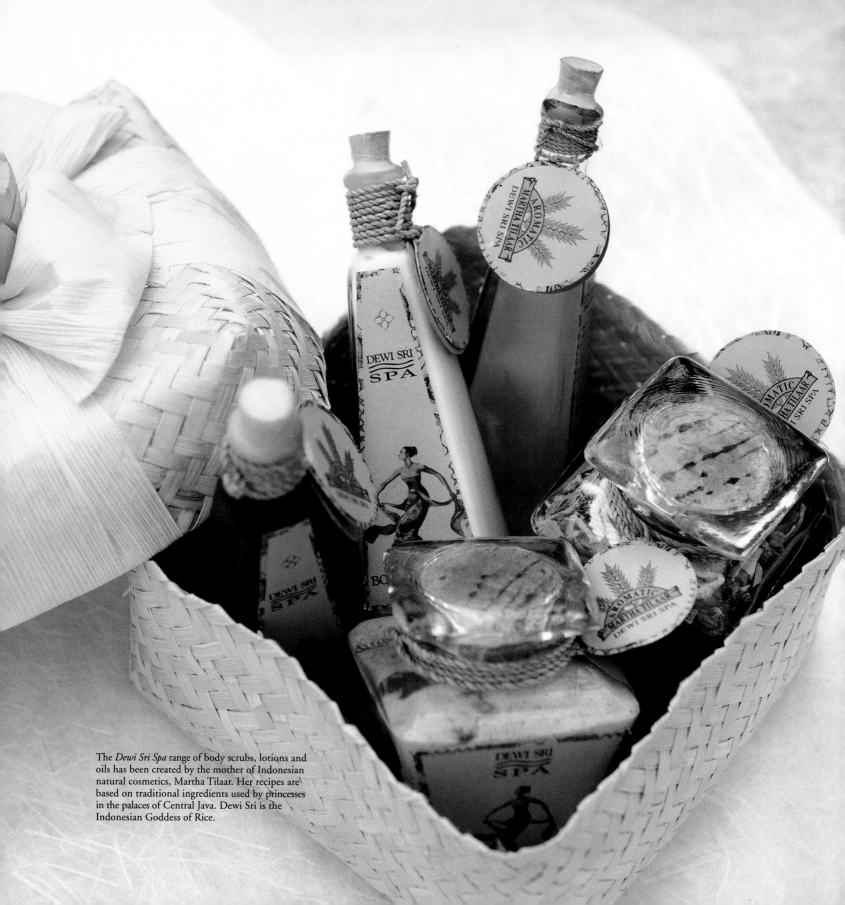

The *Dewi Sri Spa* range of body scrubs, lotions and oils has been created by the mother of Indonesian natural cosmetics, Martha Tilaar. Her recipes are based on traditional ingredients used by princesses in the palaces of Central Java. Dewi Sri is the Indonesian Goddess of Rice.

natural spa products

Wish it were not the case, but precious few of us can visit a tropical spa, all of the time. But we can relive just a whiff of the experience back home. Asian-based companies and some of the spas themselves have rummaged through nature's botanical store cupboard to create body scrubs, massage blends, essential oils and skin lotions redolent of the exotic. Not only do the aromas and textures of these products transport our souls to a tropical paradise, their natural content makes them suitable for all skin types. Here are some of the best tropical spa products available.

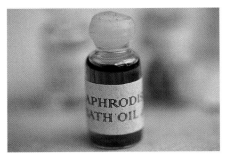

The small range of *Aphrodisia Massage Oils* is designed to do what its name suggests. Asian people understand that massage is all about sensual healing for the emotions as well as for the body; these oils are based on such exotic tropical blooms as jasmine, gardenia and champak.

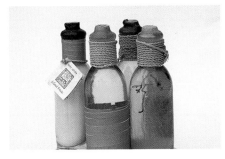

The entire range of *Esens* products – from massage oils to skin preparations – has been lovingly concocted by spa consultants Cary and Kim Collier who have spent years researching the natural health remedies of Indonesia. These aromatic lotions and potions are popular among Asian destination spas.

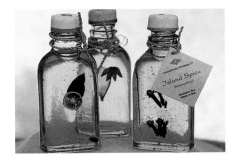

Mandara Spa is one of Asia's foremost spa companies, taking its name from the Mandara . of Balinese legend – a mythical mountain that flows with eternal youth. This should be incentive enough to purchase some of their highly effective range of *Mandara Massage Oils.*

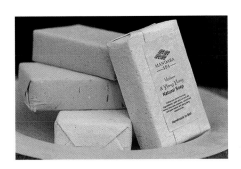

The *Mandara Soaps* from the *Mandara Spa* company come in such exotic flavours as Patchouli and Mandarin, Coffee and Pumice, Clove and Nutmeg and Goat's Milk and Canaga. They are wonderfully packaged in hand-made paper.

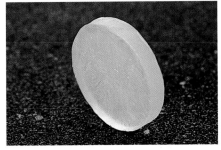

The *Personalized Spa & Resort* range of products are 100 percent natural and handmade. The company specializes in producing natural soaps, lotions, scrubs and aromatic massage oils with ingredients such as Goat's Milk and Lavender.

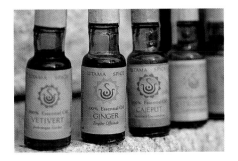

In addition to running weekend workshops aimed at reawakening the female sensual spirit, *Naz Workshops* is the distributor for *Utama Spice*, an Ubud-based company producing a range of authentic essential oils from the Spice Islands.

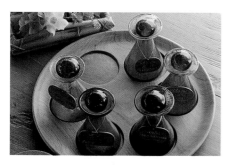

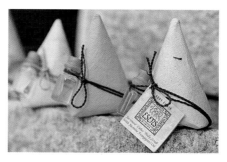

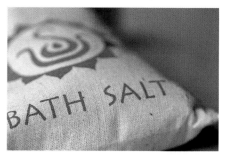

The very names of the massage oils from the *Spa at Bali Hyatt* – Stargaze, Moonlight, Spirit – are enough to transport you from the confines of your bathroom to a tropical shoreline, a good enough reason to invest in a few bottles for life in the city. The quality of these oils is superlative and they are packaged in hand-crafted ceramics and bottles.

Traditional body scrubs from *Esens* come with a one-shot massage oil. The Javanese *lulur*, for example, is a spice and yoghurt exfoliation and body polishing process. It is traditionally used by Javanese women prior to their wedding day. Now the aromatic experience can be enjoyed by everyone either as a spa treatment or packaged as a powder to take home.

The *Utama Spice* range of bath salts combines coarse sea salt crystals, harvested from the Balinese coast, with potent essential oils. A salt bath is a wonderful body detox; it relies on the nutrients in the salt to draw out toxins from the body. It also acts as an exfoliator for the skin, leaving it feeling soft and smooth.

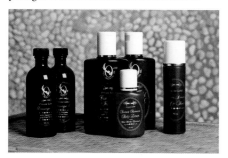

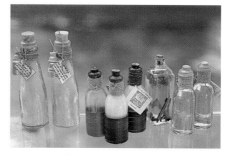

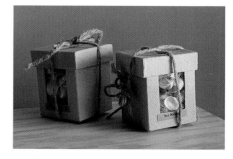

This range of body products are as 'super deluxe' as the spa from which they hail. *The Oriental Spa*'s own body creams and oils have both a rich texture and aroma and are made under licence exclusively. In the realm of beauty, friends back home could not wish for a better surprise gift. And they look attractive with dark blue packaging and spa logo.

Part of the attraction of body products from Asia is their packaging which makes of use of local materials to produce an ethnic look. Hand-blown glass, hand-made recycled paper, cork, wax, twine and even shells are transformed creatively by local hands, to add to the 'must-have' appeal of natural body foods.

As well as body products, some tropical spa shops sell gift items with an irresistible flavour of the exotic. Available exclusively at the *Nusa Dua Spa*, this box contains seashells that are harvested from the waters of the Java Sea, Indian Ocean and the famously deep Lombok Strait all of which encircle the island of Bali.

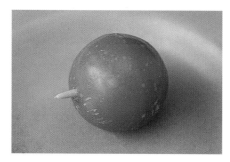

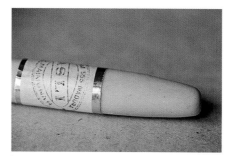

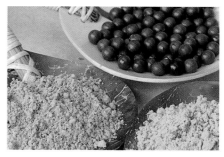

Indonesian *jamu* comes in all sorts of weird and wonderful forms with all sorts of prescriptions. Inside this waxy bomb is an explosion of potent spices to enhance male virility. The contents are dissolved in warm water and drunk. Contact Jeannine at *Jamu Traditional Spa*, KulKul Bali Resort, Kuta for some of the more unusual varieties.

The famous *tongkat* from the Indonesian island of Madura is an essential element in every woman's vanity case. This tampon-like stick is inserted into the vagina for a few minutes. It absorbs moisture and so shrinks the orifice. It is used before sex. It is washed and left to dry naturally so that it can be used time and again.

Mustika Ratu, one of Indonesia's natural beauty companies, offers over 60 *jamu* products to enhance health and beauty. Natural ingredients, formulated for specific needs, are available in powder or pill form or simply as a cocktail of dried herbs. They are ingested. The most popular *jamus* are devised for slimming and for increasing vitality and virility.

Resource Directory

The products listed on pages 172–174 are available at the outlets listed below. If they are credited to a particular spa, they will be available exclusively from that spa (please refer to spa directory on right).

Dewi Sri Spa products available from:
Martha Tilaar, Puri Ayu Martha Tilaar,
Jalan Pulokambing 11/1, Kawasan Industri Pulogadung,
Jakarta 13930, Indonesia
tel (62) 21 460 3717 fax (62) 21 460 6246

Esens products are available from:
PT Putrindo Mekar Sejati, Siligita, Permata Blok V/10,
Nusa Dua, Bali 80363, Indonesia
tel/fax (62) 361 771 991
email Collierspas@hotmail.com

Utama Spice oils are available from *Nazli Anwari* at:
Naz Workshops, 8B Stevens Close, Singapore 257948
tel (65) 2359329 fax (65) 7328223
email Nazli@earthcorp.com

Mandara Spa products are available from spas operated by *Mandara Spa* and from:
Mandara Spa, PO Box 1125, Denpasar 80000,
Bali, Indonesia
tel (62) 361 755 572 fax (62) 361 755 573
email jmatthews@mandaraspa.com

Mustika Ratu products are available at:
Mustika Ratu, Graha Mustika Ratu, PH Floor, Jalan Gotot
Subroto Kav. 74–75, Jakarta 12870, Indonesia
tel (62) 21 830 6745–59 fax (62) 21 830 6753

Personalized Spa & Resort range is available from
Joanne Feinstein at:
241 Lafayette Avenue, Dicky Brook Farm, Cortlandt
Manor, New York 10566, USA
tel/fax (1) 914 736 0030
website http://www.styleworks.com

Weekend retreats are organized by:
Breathing Space, 39 Tras Street, Singapore 078976
tel (65) 2203867 fax (65) 2236216
email admin@breathingspace.com.sg
website http//www.breathingspace.com.sg

Erotic Women's Workshops are organized by
Nazli Anwari, see above.
Naz Workshops (see above)

Spa Directory

Banyan Tree Phuket, 33 Moo 4 Srisoonthorn Road,
Cherngtalay, Amphur Talang, Phuket 83110, Thailand
tel (66) 76 324374 fax (66) 76 324375
email phuket@banyantree.com

Banyan Tree Bintan, Site A4, Lagoi, Bintan Island,
Indonesia
tel (62) 771 26918/19 fax (62) 771 81348
email bintan@banyantree.com

Begawan Giri Estate, PO Box 54, Ubud 80571, Indonesia
tel (62) 361 978888 fax (62) 361 978889
email admin@begawan.com

The Chedi, Desa Melinggih Kelod Payangan,
Gianyar 80572, Bali, Indonesia
tel (62) 361 975963 fax (62) 361 975968
email chediubd@ghmhotels.com
http://www.ghmhotels.com

Chiva-Som International Health Resort,
73/4 Petchkasem Road, Hua Hin 77110, Thailand
tel (66) 32 536536 fax (66) 32 511154

The Datai, Jalan Teluk Datai, 07000 Pulau Langkawi,
Kedah Darul Aman, Malaysia
tel (60) 4 9592500 fax (60) 4 9592600

Four Seasons Resort Bali at Jimbaran Bay
Jimbaran, Denpasar 80361, Bali, Indonesia
tel (62) 361 701010 fax (62) 361 701020
email Belinda.Sheperd@fourseasons.com

Four Seasons Resort Bali at Sayan,
Sayan, Ubud, Gianyar 80571, Bali, Indonesia
tel (62) 361 977 577 fax (62) 361 977 588
email Belinda.Sheperd@fourseasons.com

The Bali Hyatt, PO Box 392, Sanur, Bali, Indonesia
tel (62) 361 281234 fax (62) 361 287693
email bhyatt@dps.mega.net.id

The Ibah, Tjampuhan, Ubud, Bali, Indonesia
tel (62) 361 974466 fax (62) 361 974467
email ibah@denpasar.wasantara.net.id

Jamu Body Treatments, Jalan Cipete VIII, 82A, Cipete,
Jakarta Selatan, Indonesia
tel (62) 21 765 9691 fax (62) 21 765 9693

Jamu Traditional Spa, KulKulBali, PO Box 3097, Denpasar
80030, Bali, Indonesia
tel (62) 361 752520 fax (62) 361 752519

email kulkul@indosat.net.id
Javana Spa, PT Sarana Prima Budaya Raga,
Plaza Bisnis Kemang 2, Jalan Kemang Raya No 2,
Jakarta Selatan 12730, Indonesia
tel (62) 21 719 8327 fax (62) 21 719 5555

Le Meridien Nirwana Golf and Spa Resort, PO Box 158,
Tabanan, Bali, Indonesia
tel (62) 361 815900 fax (62) 361 815901/07

Moana Spa, Turi Beach Resort, Batam, Indonesia
tel (62) 778 761080 fax (62) 778 761043

Nikko Bali Resort and Spa, Jalan Raya Nusa Dua Selatan,
Nusa Dua 80363, Bali, Indonesia
tel (62) 361 773377 fax (62) 361 773388
email sales@nikkobali.com

Novotel Coralia Lombok Mandalika Resort,
Pantai Putri Nyale, Pujut - Lombok Tengah, Indonesia
tel (62) 370 653333 fax (62) 370 653555
email Novotel@lombokonline.com

Nusa Dua Beach Hotel & Spa, PO Box 1028,
Denpasar, Bali, Indonesia
tel (62) 361 771210 fax (62) 361 772621
email ndbhnet@indosat.net.id

The Oriental Bangkok, 48 Oriental Avenue,
Bangkok 10500, Thailand
tel (66) 2 2360400 (hotel); (66) 2 4397613/4 (spa)
fax (66) 2 2361937/9 (hotel); (66) 2 4397587 (spa)

Hotel Padma Bali, Jalan Padma no 1, Legian,
PO Box 1107 TBB, Bali, Indonesia
tel (62) 361 752111 fax (62) 361 752140

Pita Maha Resort, Jalan Sanggingan, PO Box 198,
Ubud 80571, Bali, Indonesia
tel (62) 361 974330 fax (62) 361 974329
email pitamaha@dps.mega.net.id

The Serai, Buitan, PO Box 13, Karangasem 80871,
Bali, Indonesia
tel (62) 363 41011 fax (62) 363 41015
email seraimanggis@ghmhotels.com
http://www.ghmhotels.com

St Gregory Javana Spa, Hotel Plaza Parkroyal,
7500A Beach Road, Singapore 199591
tel (65) 298001 fax (65) 2908083
email plazahtl@mbox2singnet.com.sg

Tugu Hotel, Jalan Pantai Batu Bolong, Desa Canggu,
Canggu Beach, Bali, Indonesia
tel (62) 361 731701/3 fax (62) 361 731 704
email bali@tuguhotels.com

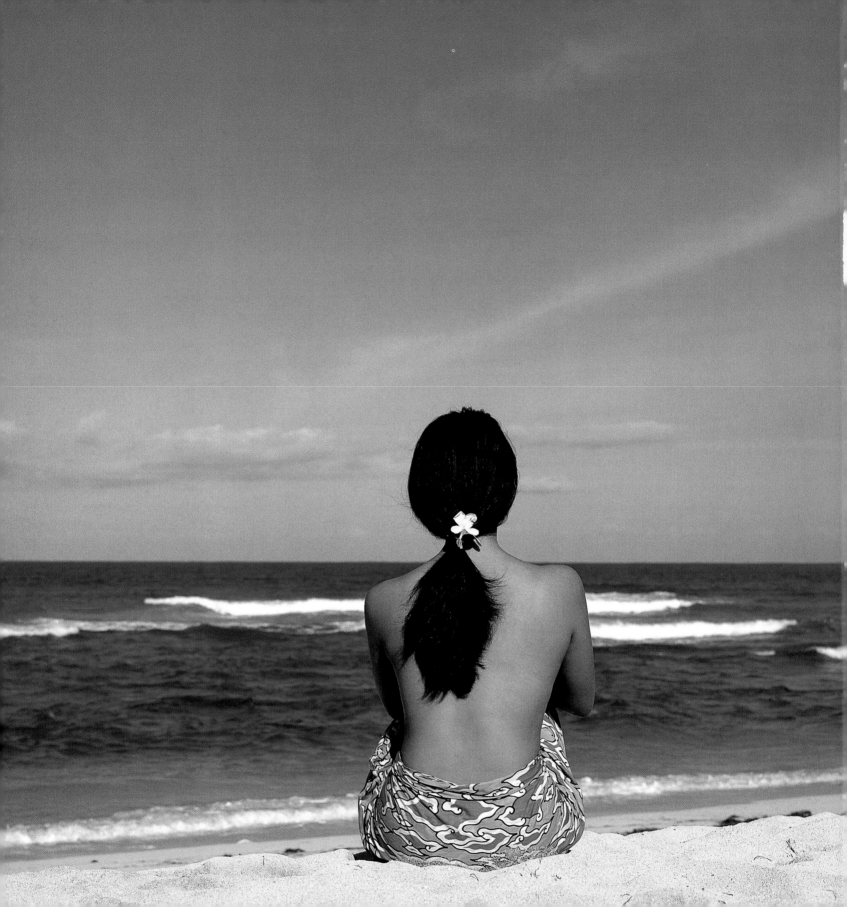

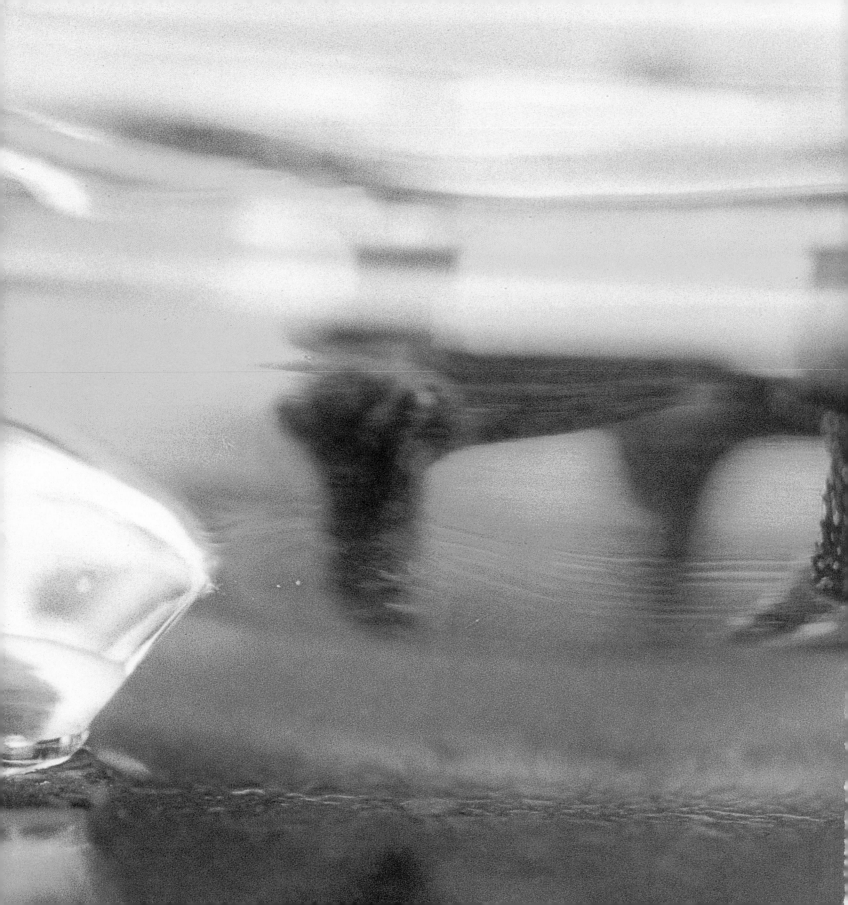